Pilgrim Souls

For Pat and
Otto
With affection
Jim Oct 29/14

Pilgrim Souls

Caring for a Loved One with Dementia

Jim Lotz

Formac Publishing Company Limited
Halifax

Copyright © 2013 by Jim Lotz
All interior photos are the property of the author.

All rights reserved. No part of this book may be reproduced or transmitted in
any form or by any means, electronic or mechanical, including photocopying,
or by any information storage or retrieval system, without permission in
writing from the publisher.

Formac Publishing Company Limited recognizes the support of the Province
of Nova Scotia through the Department of Communities, Culture and
Heritage. We are pleased to work in partnership with the province to develop
and promote our culture resources for all Nova Scotians. We acknowledge
the financial support of the Government of Canada through the Canada
Book Fund for our publishing activities. We acknowledge the support of the
Canada Council for the Arts which last year invested $157 million to bring
the arts to Canadians throughout the country.

 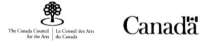

Cover design: Tyler Cleroux
Cover image: Shutterstock

Library and Archives Canada Cataloguing in Publication

Lotz, Jim, 1929-, author
    Pilgrim souls : caring for a loved one with dementia / Jim Lotz.

  ISBN 978-1-4595-0276-5 (pbk.)

        1. Lotz, Pat--Mental health. 2. Lotz, Jim, 1929- --Marriage.
3. Dementia--Patients--Family relationships--Canada. 4. Dementia--
Patients--Canada--Biography. I. Title.

RC521.L68 2013   362.196'83   C2013-904355-1

Formac Publishing Company Limited
5502 Atlantic Street
Halifax, NS, Canada
B3H 1G4
www.formac.ca

Printed and bound in Canada.

To the memory of my beloved wife and best friend,
Patricia Ann Lotz

October 20, 1930–February 13, 2012

How many loved your moments of glad grace,
And loved your beauty with love false or true,
But one man loved the pilgrim soul in you,
And loved the sorrows of your changing face.

W. B. Yeats, *"When You Are Old"*

Contents

Introduction

I seem to have loved you in numberless forms,
numberless times, in life after life, in age after age
forever… Clad in the light of a polestar piercing
the darkness of time: You become an image of what
is remembered forever.

Rabindranath Tagore, *"Manasi"*

This book tells of a love affair that dementia could not
damage or destroy.

Pat and I met and married in Montreal in 1959. We had a
wonderful, passionate, tumultuous life in that city, in Ottawa,
Vancouver, the Yukon, Scotland, England, Italy, Victoria,
rural Nova Scotia and Halifax, where we settled in 1973.

As the new century opened, Pat, aged seventy, experienced problems with her short-term memory. We dismissed
them as a normal part of aging. On August 6, 2002,
Dr. Deanna Swinemar, our family physician, tested Pat's

attention, memory and language and found no problems. At the Memory Disability Clinic on August 10, 2006, Pat was diagnosed with "cognitive impairment no dementia" (CIND). By July 2007, Pat had lost her short-term memory. Despite this, our life together proceeded quite normally and we enjoyed plenty of love and laughter.

On October 19, 2009, Dr. Laurie Mallery at the Memory Disability Clinic tested Pat's cognitive abilities and concluded that she had "severe (end-stage) Alzheimer dementia" that required "total care for activities of daily living and constant twenty-four-hour supervision." I became Pat's main caregiver, with the help of home support workers from the Canadian Red Cross.

Pat fell on Saturday, February 11, 2012, while I was on respite.

Taken to the emergency department of the Halifax Infirmary, she was x-rayed and nothing wrong was found. After a night in hospital, she came home with me and slept peacefully. On the following Monday, with Pat obviously in pain, I took her back to the emergency department. She died there at 11:25 p.m. on the eve of Saint Valentine's Day from causes unrelated to dementia.

On October 20, 2011, *The Nova Scotian*, the Sunday insert in the Halifax *Chronicle Herald*, ran my article on how Pat and I coped with her dementia. Headed "Now where's that toothpaste?" it attracted a great deal of attention and positive feedback. In an accompanying piece, Dr. Ken Rockwood, a professor of geriatric medicine at Dalhousie University, wrote, "Dementia will become more common." He added that my "candid account" of how Pat and I dealt with it "offers us lessons about science, society and life." He concluded, "Mr. Lotz's tough example shows how people can triumph, even in tragedy."

This book tells the story of our lives, identifying how our relationship influenced the way we dealt with Pat's dementia. Pat, the kindest of beings, would want me to share our story, to give hope and comfort to others.

Family doctors know little about disorders of the mind, in part because of their complexity — all those billions of neurons and synapses! — and in part because they see patients in offices or clinics and know little of their lives. A doctor saw a patient with dementia and decided she had no problems: "She has just come back from a holiday in Europe with her husband." The woman's husband had been dead for twenty years and she had never been to Europe.

When a loved one is diagnosed with dementia, it is normal for those closest to them to become fearful, alarmed, anxious and fall prey to despair. A woman whose husband developed Alzheimer's compared life with him to "being chained to a corpse." Sufferers are still human beings and need love, support and comfort more than ever. In time, those who care for them, and about them, learn to cope with the sudden and unpredictable changes that take place as the disease worsens, and life can be surprisingly normal.

Pat would ask me, "Who are you?" I'd smile and reply, "The guy who loves you and looks after you" or "Jim" or "Your ever-loving husband."

She might not know who I was, but I knew who she was. And that was all that really mattered.

A caregiver told me, "You always treated your wife as your wife and always showed your love." Friends commented on how "heroic" and "noble" and "faithful" I was in caring for Pat, calling her "a burden," referring to my "ordeal." I never saw my role or my experiences in caring for my beloved wife in those terms. What else could I do for this beautiful, spirited woman I adored, the alpha and omega of my life, whom I loved from the first moment I saw her, who had so enriched my being, to whom I had made a solemn vow of "pure and endless love" when I took her to be "my wedded wife...for better or worse, for richer or poorer, in sickness and in health, to love and to cherish"?

The first two stanzas of Roy Croft's poem "Love" express how I felt about Pat:

> *I love you*
> *Not only for what you are,*
> *But for what I am*
> *When I am with you.*

> *I love you,*
> *Not only for what*
> *You have made of yourself,*
> *But for what*
> *You are making of me.*

Pat and I did not have a perfect marriage, for, as the old saying puts it, "Perfection is the enemy of the good." We argued and we almost split up several times. Yet, we had a very good marriage and a wonderful relationship, almost to Pat's last day. What would have become of me had I not married Pat, I cannot say. But my life could not have been more rich, rewarding and interesting than it was with the remarkable woman I married. Through joys and sorrows, through rows and reconciliations, through periods of depression and times of sheer exhilaration, our love for each other flowered, strengthened and deepened.

Brought up in the British tradition of reserve and reticence in emotional matters, we seldom displayed our love for each other in public. Yet, friends, and even strangers, recognized how well attuned to each other we were. A friend wrote that she'd "noticed how you both interacted and your love and respect for one another just shone!" A caregiver wrote, "You both made me realize how powerful love is. Thank you for touching my life."

As best friends, we always did what we did for each other without thought of return. This became a vital factor in caring for Pat as she sank deeper and deeper into dementia. I am sure that Pat knew that I was there for her, caring for her with unreserved love, maintaining the friendly relationship we had always had, that unbreakable bond between us that dementia could not destroy. Even in the depths of Pat's affliction, we had many moments of glad grace that banished sorrows from her face with joy and laughter.

Caring for a person with dementia is not simply a medical matter. It's a management one, requiring the setting of goals, the identification of strategies to enable you and the sufferer to live as normal a life as possible and endless attention to tactics to help to achieve that goal. However, something more than this is needed. Caregivers must know themselves, their limits and capabilities, as the behaviour of the afflicted person changes from day to day, sometimes from moment to moment. Flotsam and jetsam from the past surfaces, good and bad memories of times together emerge, old wounds open and you are tested to your uttermost limits.

I have not sugarcoated my shortcomings, failings, mistakes and sheer stupidity in caring for Pat, things I should not have done, words I should not have spoken. Pat had ever been a forgiving person and that did not change during her dementia. Try as I did to make our life together as normal as possible, the demons of despair, hopelessness and anxiety swooped down on me from time to time. I struggled to avoid becoming a victim or a martyr, to retreat into self-pity and lose myself in guilt and recrimination. I became acutely aware of my shortcomings as I struggled, every day and in every way, to infuse with love everything I did for Pat and with Pat.

There is but one constant thing, one guiding light in caring for someone with dementia, and that is love. Fortunately, by the time Pat developed dementia, our love for each other had become rock solid, enduring, the pillar of our lives. As St. Paul wrote to the Corinthians two thousand years ago, he was nothing without love. Nor were Pat and I. As I recall our life together, before and after she developed dementia, Paul's words come to me with startling clarity:

> Love is patient, love is kind. It does not envy, it does not boast, it is not proud.
> It is not rude, it is not self-seeking, it is not easily angered, it keeps no record of wrongs.
> Love does not delight in evil but rejoices with the truth.
> It always protects, always trusts, always hopes, always perseveres.

And, most of all, as I learned through my life with Pat, "Love never fails."

This book consists of two parts.

"Background: Life Before Dementia" tells how I met Pat, describes our lives before that magical moment and outlines our family backgrounds. A chapter deals with our careers, travel and the lifelong learning in which we engaged, each in our own way. Another chapter covers our emotional relationships and how they developed through our married life.

"Foreground: The Long Goodbye" describes the progress of Pat's dementia and how we coped with it.

Pat and I never considered ourselves as other than ordinary people. We found, in Canada, opportunities for personal development and service to others that we could never have dreamed of growing up in working-class Britain in the grim war and postwar years. By sharing our story, we hope to inspire, help and give strength to those caring for loved ones with dementia and other disabling conditions.

PART ONE
Background: Life Before Dementia

By understanding the person's personality, life experiences, support systems and ways of coping, the individual's physical, social, emotional and spiritual needs can be met.

Day to Day, Alzheimer Society, August 2002

Alzheimer's, a progressive, degenerative disease, slowly but surely destroys vital brain cells, blotting our memory, changing behaviour, making every day a challenge for those caring for sufferers. Every dementia is different because every sufferer is different. They live in a very immediate present, with no short-term memory but some long-term memory in some cases. As Oliver Sacks notes in *Musicophilia*, "…aspects of one's essential character, of personality and personhood, of self, survive — along with certain, almost indestructible forms of memory — even in very advanced dementia."

Our character, and much of our behaviour, is formed early in life by forces of which we are only dimly aware. As we age and memories pile up, the narrative of our lives includes dreams, urges, unresolved issues, things we did that we should not have done, achievements that enriched our lives, interactions with others, disturbing and reassuring. Ghosts from the past become very real presences.

Our lifelong passion for each other made it relatively easy to care for Pat. I tried hard to understand my past and how it conditioned my behaviour and to recall what I had learned about Pat that would help me in caring for her. At times, she seemed to be almost a stranger to me, at others warm and responsive, an ideal companion.

Renoir claimed we should see ourselves like corks floating down a stream, letting the water take us where it will. We move forwards in life. But we can only understand who we are by looking backwards, upstream, figuring out when we moved swiftly and the times we ended up in backwaters or stagnant pools. We try to identify what helped or hindered the smooth flow of our lives. Dealing with a person with dementia forces you to confront yourself — and the loved one — at the very roots of your being. You come to know yourself, and that person, in ways never before possible when life was normal, stable and foreseeable. In caring for someone you love, you learn to be creative and imaginative in meeting your own physical, emotional and spiritual needs.

Life becomes difficult.

But never dull!

Chapter One
My Lucky Break

Somewhere there waiteth in this world of ours
For one lone soul another lonely soul,
Each chasing each through all the weary hours
And meeting strangely at one sudden goal.

Edwin Arnold, *"Somewhere"*

Pat and I met by accident.

Or, more correctly, because of an accident.

In February 1959, I sat in an upstairs office in the Arctic Institute of North America in Montreal, preparing to go with an expedition to the ice shelf of Northern Ellesmere Island. For no reason I can determine, a phrase from a poem buzzed around in my head, something about "time's wingéd chariot," but I could not place the source.

In search of it, I descended the stairs to the institute's

library. Out of the corner of my eye, I caught sight of a stranger, a woman in a blue sweater and grey skirt, leaning over a card catalogue.

That moment stays in my memory as if it happened yesterday.

"Anyone know the poem that has something about 'time's wingéd chariot' in it?" I asked the library staff.

The woman at the card catalogue turned towards me.

And that was it — love at first sight!

Petite, neatly dressed, with an attractive white streak in her dark hair, lustrous brown eyes, a generous mouth and a strong chin, here before me stood the most beautiful woman I had ever seen.

She spoke:

> *"But at my back I always hear*
> *Time's wingéd chariot hurrying near:*
> *And yonder all before us lie*
> *Deserts of vast eternity."*

I thanked her and we introduced ourselves. She was Pat Wicks, doing her library practice. She told me the lines came from a poem by Andrew Marvell, a seventeenth-century Englishman, bent on luring his mistress — then a general term for a genteel young lady — into bed. Pat quoted the first lines of "To His Coy Mistress:"

> *Had we but world enough, and time,*
> *This coyness, lady, would be no crime.*

Did this beautiful, engaging stranger think I was using poetry to pick her up? We chatted for a while. After studying at Sir George Williams University while holding down a job, Pat had graduated with the Governor General's Medal in English, something I discovered much later in our married life. When she received her library degree, she would move to Vancouver to work in the city's public library.

We began dating.

I learned that Pat had been born in Brighton, England, and arrived in Canada in 1952 as an indentured servant looking after the children of the British trade commissioner. She also cooked, cleaned and served at table.

After two years, she quit, worked for Bell Telephone then became a library assistant at McGill University, from which I had graduated with a master's degree in geography in 1957. Just before convocation, Svenn Orvig, professor of meteorology at the university, phoned and asked if I would be interested in going on an Arctic expedition as a weather observer. Brought up on heroic tales of Peary, Scott, Shackleton, Franklin and other polar explorers, I did not hesitate to sign on with Operation Hazen, a major part of Canada's contribution to the Third International Geophysical Year, during which nations cooperated in a wide range of studies of natural phenomena in the polar region.

At midnight on April 28, I jumped out of a C-119, a Flying Boxcar, onto the surface of Lake Hazen at 81°48' N and began my career in the Arctic. I spent the summers of 1957 and 1958 on the Gilman Glacier, which drains from the interior ice cap of Northern Ellesmere Island.

I returned to Montreal in the fall of 1958, intent on settling down, finding a steady job and a suitable mate and living a normal, unadventurous life. In the hope of breaking into the writing game, I took a job selling ads for *The Montrealer* magazine.

Talking to my friend Otto about ways of meeting women, he suggested I join him on a ski trip to Val David. Here he took me to the top of a gentle slope down which I slid, losing my balance and ending up in a tangled heap at the bottom. My ankle hurt, so I staggered over to the ski hut to be fussed over by the women in our party.

Walking around Montreal the next day, trying to sell ads, my ankle pained me. With British stoicism (or stupidity) I ignored the mounting agony. After ten days without making a sale, I visited a young lady in hospital with whom I had been keeping company; she was having allergy tests. As we chatted, a member of the ski party, a nurse, arrived.

"How's the ankle?" she asked.

"Bit painful."

"You should get it x-rayed. They can do that downstairs."

I took her advice.

At eleven in the evening, I left the hospital in a wheelchair. I had broken my ankle.

And so ended my short career in ad sales.

While working up the results of my observations from the 1958 season with Operation Hazen, I had been asked if I was interested in leading an expedition to the ice shelf of Northern Ellesmere Island. The Arctic Institute of North America had a contract with the United States Air Force to determine if bombers could land there. I turned down the offer. Now incapacitated, I phoned up my contact at the institute. Was the leadership position still open? It had been filled, but the expedition needed a meteorologist with Arctic experience.

By the time the venture left, my ankle would be healed.

So I signed up to go again to the High Arctic. And met Pat.

As she and I went out together, we discovered we had much in common and enjoyed each other's company. In

April, I moved to Boston to await the C-130 that would take us to the ice shelf. Pat joined me on weekends and we recognized the lone soul in each other. We had a joyous time walking around the old parts of Boston, drinking in bars, just talking, happy in simply being together. We spent an enchanted evening watching Danny Kaye conduct the Boston Pops orchestra.

By now, I was hopelessly in love with Pat, but had no idea how she felt about me. On her last visit, I took Pat to the train for Montreal, then walked back to my hotel through a dark, dreary, windswept night, feeling a terrible sense of loss. At the hotel, I wrote a passionate letter to Pat, declaring my love and asking her to marry me.

A few days later, I was on Ward Hunt Island, which lies in the middle of the ice shelf of Northern Ellesmere Island, at the edge of the Arctic Ocean. The C-130 landed on the ice shelf, disgorged the equipment and supplies we needed then flew away. We built huts and sorted out equipment. A tractor dragged a trailer to the edge of the ice shelf where I set up a weather station. My companion and I lived there for four months.

Storms swept over our trailer and we lived in a foggy void for months on end. Quite suddenly, the fog would lift and we could see the whole coastline of Northern Ellesmere Island in all its pristine beauty, the huge mass of Rambow Hill thrusting into the ice shelf, the snow-clad peaks of the British Empire Range standing in stark relief.

Because our equipment kept breaking down, we had regular airdrops that included Pat's letters. In one of them she agreed to marry me. I was ecstatic, reading the letter again and again in our cramped quarters. Pat's decision to marry me, and her other loving letters, helped me retain my sanity throughout that long, icy summer.

After that long summer in the Arctic, the C-130 picked us up from the ice shelf in September 1959.

Pat had told me that she liked Wedgwood pottery. The BX (Base Exchange) at Thule air force base was having a sale on Wedgwood. With my usual overenthusiasm and desire to please Pat, I bought a large quantity of it. She liked small pieces of the pottery; I now had almost enough to open a restaurant.

After travelling to Washington for a debriefing, I flew to Pasadena to see Paul Walker, the glaciologist on the ice-shelf expedition. We had been good friends in Boston, haunting bookstores and buying books, sampling restaurants, going to movies, talking endlessly about the women with whom we were in love. Paul had suffered a stroke on the ice shelf and lay, paralyzed, in a bed in his parents' home. He died a few months later. We had become like brothers before we left Boston and in the early days of the expedition. I was devastated by Paul's death but determined to do something to keep his memory green in that icebound land. The Canadian Board on Geographic Names accepted my suggestion that the hill on Ward Hunt Island bear his name.

From Los Angeles, I flew to Vancouver, took a hotel room and began to write up the results of my research on the ice shelf. Pat had moved to Vancouver after graduating from library school and worked in the reference section of the central library. She and I spent as much time as possible together before I returned to Montreal to await her arrival.

We were married in the Church of St. Mark in Longueil on December 12, 1959. I retain a vivid memory of glancing sideways at Pat as we stood at the altar, utterly entranced by her beauty.

My ankle pains me from time to time. But I always refer to what happened to it as my lucky break.

Chapter Two
Before We Met

It is better to know as little as possible of the defects of the person with whom you wish to pass your life.

Jane Austen, *Pride and Prejudice*

Pat and I knew little about each other when we married.

We had both earned our living since our teens by doing a variety of menial jobs. Strong-willed, stubborn, impatient, we both had tempers and relished our independence and peculiar ways of doing things.

Pat, born in 1930, had, like me, grown up during the Second World War and the years of austerity after it. These had been grim days, when even bread was rationed.

In her younger years, Pat had visited Denmark and spent a year as an *au pair* with a doctor's family in Carcassonne in southern France. Treated as a member of the family, she recalled her time with the Soums as a wonderful episode in her life. She also became fluent in French.

Growing up in an urban setting, Pat developed a love of the countryside, fueled by her interest in romantic poets.

Born in Liverpool, England, in January 1929, I grew up there and in my mother's village of Oldmeldrum in Aberdeenshire. Had we paid attention to Disraeli's claim, Pat and I would never have married. He saw northern and southern England as two nations:

> *...between whom there is no intercourse and no sympathy, two areas ignorant of each other's habits, thoughts and feelings, as if they were dwellers in different zones or inhabitants of different planets.*

Despite what we had in common, Pat and I differed greatly in many respects because of our cultural backgrounds.

The legacy of industrialization hung over Liverpool and Manchester where I went to university. You could almost taste the air. One day the sky went black at noon because a layer of air trapped the crud under it. In our working-class area, the uniform streets replicated each other over endless stretches. A hard land and hard manual work bred hard men and a macho culture of coarseness and directness. We called a spade a spade — or a bloody shovel.

Southerners grew up in less polluted places. Here, in rural areas and small towns and cities like Brighton, a more genteel way of life prevailed. I told Pat that the north made the wealth of Britain and the people in the south spent it.

She liked stories and books with happy endings and disliked conflict. I loved challenges, new experiences and opportunities to try new ways of solving problems.

Growing up in Liverpool, my cultural baggage included a strong, sometimes warped, sense of humour. The city spawned comics, including Tommy Handley. When a cat strolled on stage during one of his stand-up routines, he shooed it away, saying, "This is a monologue, not a catalogue." During the war, this Liverpudlian kept up the spirits of the British with *ITMA* (*It's That Man Again*), a politically incorrect, madcap radio programme featuring topical gags, agonizing one-liners, surreal storylines and ambiguous catchphrases like "Can I do you now, sir?"

Pat and I relished the absurdist British humour pioneered by Edward Lear and Lewis Carroll and continued by the Monty Python gang. We enjoyed the Goons:

> *Eccles: When you're dead, people are going to look up to you.*
>
> *Neddy Seagoon, flattered and flustered: Why?*
>
> *Eccles: We're going to bury you in a tree.*

Even as dementia clouded her mind, Pat retained her sense of humour.

The cheerful cheekiness of the Beatles, which I share, stems from their Liverpool roots, as does their dislike of authority and extempore manner of speaking. These qualities arose from the sense that Liverpudlians have of being outsiders. John Lennon recalled, "We were the ones that were looked down upon as animals by southerners." To be a northerner, tough and uncultured, was one thing. But to also be a "scouse," named for one of the main dishes we Liverpudlians ate, placed you at the lowest levels of British society.

And so we developed thick skins, chips on our shoulders and aggressiveness along with our sense of humour. Properly channeled, this gave us great energy and drive. However, when I became involved in community development, colleagues accused me of "coming on too strong," a dangerous thing to do in a post-colonial nation with people known for being polite and deferential to authority.

Among her many other gifts to me, Pat helped me to deal with my aggressive impulses. I always wanted to solve problems, rather than study or talk about them. This dumb male attitude placed severe strains on our relationship at times.

Growing up in the British working class, Pat and I absorbed aspects of its culture: common sense, independence — you should never be beholden to others — the belief that you had to work for what you got, dislike of pretense and pomposity (people getting above themselves, *au-dessus de leur gare*, as we joked) and egalitarianism based on an abhorrence of the class system that cribbed, cabined and confined so many people in Britain, stifling their potential.

Working-class people feel they are being continually judged by those who believe they are their betters. As a result, they tend to judge themselves, often much too harshly. In a diary, Pat wrote of her feelings of low self-esteem and a lack of confidence. I could never understand why this beautiful, intelligent woman felt this way. Did Pat's feelings of inadequacy arise from something in her childhood — or from the barrage of advertising that tells modern women what they should look like, how they should run their lives, what they should wear, and more? Whatever the cause, the feelings sent Pat on a spiritual quest that led to "the sorrows of [her] changing face," one of the many things about her that I loved. My quest to transcend my working-class background turned me outwards, ever ready to try new things, take risks to prove myself to myself and others.

Pat and I survived the German blitzes on our cities. How this shaped our characters and destinies I have no way of knowing. But we always felt happy to have survived, to be alive.

In April 1942, Hitler, infuriated by attacks by British bombers on the historic cities of Rostock and Lubeck, ordered raids on British cities with buildings listed as cultural attractions in the Baedeker guidebooks. They included Bath.

Pat's father worked for the British Admiralty during the war. It evacuated half its staff to the "safe" city of Bath, which had no military installations. On April 25 and 26, German bombers of Luftflotte III attacked the city, destroying or damaging beyond repair over a thousand houses, killing 417 people but leaving listed buildings untouched.

A firebomb hit the Wicks's flat; the family lost all its possessions, including Pat's teddy bear. Pat's mother, Rosamond, wrote to our daughter, Annette, "Teddy had been given to me when I was five years old, he was my treasure and, in time, became the most treasured possession of Pat, the eldest daughter… He had listened to her baby talk, and, later, to her childish confidences — and most of all, he was always there when she was in trouble (as she so often was!)."

It's hard to tell how a single incident influences a life. Apparently Teddy survived the fire, but Pat did not dare to enter the gutted flat to recover him. She often told me she was a coward, perhaps because of her failure to rescue her beloved companion. I told her that everyone is a coward about something; I'm scared stiff of heights. This did nothing to assuage her guilt about abandoning Teddy.

Liverpool, my hometown, had been the target of sporadic

German raids in the first two years of the war. From May 2 to 8, 1941, the Luftwaffe concentrated its fury on the city. We went to bed in the shelter in our front room, wondering if we would wake up in the morning.

I still remember the characteristic pulsating throb of the engines of the German bomber as it roared towards our house, loosing its bombs. Then came a mighty explosion as one fell behind the house next door. The bomb stripped our roof, blew out windows and turned our backyard wall into rubble. Firefighters hauling hoses through our living room and kitchen added to the damage.

Another danger then confronted us as the houses next door caught fire and flames roared out of their windows. Fortunately, we were separated from them by a passageway, a jigger or howler in the local argot. The fire next door did not reach our house. Six neighbours, whose names we never knew, died in the inferno. They were buried in a mass grave. We cleaned up the house and went on with our lives.

Neither Pat's family nor mine ever had much money. We became accustomed to living frugally, keeping out of debt, refusing to rely on the never-never (buying stuff on credit). Austerity, during and after the war, reinforced these habits. We wasted little in our home and had no interest in consuming conspicuously. Pat, a gifted seamstress, made her own wedding dress.

Our generation was not cradled in beliefs of entitlement and instant gratification. The working class in Britain learned that there is no point in complaining about problems because no one will do anything about them. Its members expected little from life — and the government — and recognized they would have to struggle for anything they needed.

These feelings faded somewhat during the war, when a tremendous sense of community and commitment to the good of others emerged. During the war, the British were better fed than before it and the number of mental disorders decreased. Amid the destruction, suffering and dislocations of the war, we made the best of what little we had.

This attitude had much to do with the way we dealt with Pat's dementia.

The war gave us another heritage that we shared, feelings of hope and a belief in a better world. No one talked about human rights or social justice; we saw them as normal aspects of life and human decency that you practised in your relationships with others. Bombs fell on the rich and the poor, the powerful and the oppressed. We learned that we are all equal in our capacity to suffer and to endure. We looked forward to a new world when the war ended in 1945 and the Labour government took power and launched the Welfare State.

It was not to be. The late 1940s and early 1950s proved to be drab and depressing without the binding forces of selflessness, service and community that marked the war years. Greyness pervaded our lives, in part because paint had been unobtainable during the war.

I had one burning ambition while growing up — to escape from my hometown and travel to distant places. I did well in high school before being conscripted into the Royal Air Force in 1947, just after my eighteenth birthday. I enjoyed basic training, which involved learning how to kill people with various weapons as well as my hands, but I was assigned to train as a radio fitter, a trade for which I was totally unsuited. I may have been dyslexic — I could never tell my left hand from my right — or just naturally clumsy.

I failed the theory and workshop exams twice before being pushed on to the next part of the course, which dealt with radio equipment. Almost as clueless at the end of the course as I had been at the beginning, I became an instructor. My time in the RAF marked the start of a lifelong suspicion of, and incompetence with, technology.

Despite acquiring two degrees in geography — or maybe because of this — I developed a terrible, faulty sense of direction that infuriated Pat. I led her astray in Pisa when I took a wrong turn and we ended up in a featureless part of the city. And there was the time we walked along the Ardentine walls of Rome when I lost my way. For me, the journey, not the arrival, has always been the goal of travel — a sentiment Pat did not share.

After graduating with a degree in geography from Manchester University in 1952, I spent the summer on the RAF reserve near Dunbar, grouse beating in the Scottish Highlands and living in a luxury hotel in London while taking a three-week course to become a manager with the United Africa Company; the Unilever subsidiary controlled much of the produce and merchandise trade on the west coast of Africa.

I did all sorts of managerial things in Kano, Katsina and Sokoto in Northern Nigeria. While stationed in Kano in May 1953, I was sworn in as a special constable, along with other whites, when riots broke out between northerners and southerners. We did what we could to stop the looting and the killing, and that was far too little.

With three other UAC managers, I rescued an African man from a mob about to murder him. As the saying goes, you can postpone the moment of truth, but you can't avoid it. The Kano riots made me realize I was working in a dying colonial order for a company interested only in profit. So I quit and returned to England.

Jobs for geographers, unless you became a teacher, were scarce in Britain in 1954. I was hired to work in a factory, then fired when the management discovered I had a university degree. I decided that if I could not find a decent job six months after returning from Africa, I would immigrate to Canada. And that is what I did. Why did I choose Canada? It was close enough to Britain that if things didn't work out, I could come back home. One of my uncles had done well in Alberta. His son, a bomber pilot with the Royal Canadian Air Force, stayed with us between missions. We found him friendly, affable and relaxed despite his dangerous trade. And an immigration officer assured me that Canada was "a great big country, growing up all over."

Pat came to Canada with a family as part of her job as a servant. She often spoke, before and during her dementia, about going back to Britain. I chose Canada and had no urge to return to "the old country." We returned several times to Britain, and Pat realized that it was not the country she had left. But she still hankered to return there, even as her memory faded.

Like many other British immigrants, I planned to go to Toronto. A dock strike in New York diverted the liner to Halifax where I landed at Pier 21. Taking a train to Ottawa, I sought work with the federal government, only to learn that I would have to be in Canada for five years before I could be hired.

My first year in Canada proved to be most inauspicious.

I found a job with Canadian Aero Services assembling mosaics of air photos. I fell asleep while being shown how to use a new piece of equipment and was fired.

After an English colleague assured me that to be a true Canadian I had to own a car, I bought a Morris Oxford, a lemon with a faulty starter, the only hand-cranked car in Ottawa. After learning to drive on my friend's huge Humber Pullman, I'd secured a provisional license. Driving home after being fired, I eased into a downtown intersection. I hit a car… or it hit me. The details of the collision remain vague in my memory. I was thrown through the door as my car tried to climb a stop sign. I had been doing a lot of judo, so rolled and emerged unscathed save for a large bruise on my thigh.

My next job involved billing stores supplied by IGA, a grocery wholesaler, a boring and monotonous task. From here I moved, after another car accident, to Freiman's, a department store in central Ottawa, as an advertising copywriter.

With poor eyesight and a tendency for my mind to wander while I was behind the wheel, plus my poor physical coordination, it became obvious to me that I was a menace on the road. Cars had not been part of Pat's life in England. She showed no interest in learning to drive or in acquiring a family vehicle. So we walked — a lot — and that had a bearing on how we coped with Pat's dementia.

After a year in dead-end jobs, I realized I would get nowhere without a Canadian university degree. I contacted the geography departments at the University of Toronto and McGill to determine what support they had for graduate students. Ken Hare, the entrepreneurial head of the latter institution, offered me a summer job as a weather observer at the McGill Subarctic Research Lab at Knob Lake in central Ungava. It paid enough to cover my university fees. During the winters I worked at the observatory on the McGill campus for $125 a month, net $116.

In 1956, I returned to Knob Lake to do the fieldwork for my master's thesis. It dealt with soils and agriculture in central Labrador. There was almost none of the former and no possibility of the latter, but I secured my second degree in geography in 1957 and became hooked on Canada's north. This led me to Operation Hazen and to that fateful day in Montreal when I went in search of a quotation from a seventeenth-century English poet and met the love of my life.

Chapter Three
Families

They fuck you up, your mum and dad.
They may not mean to, but they do.
They fill you with the faults they had
And add some extra, just for you.

Philip Larkin, *This Be the Verse*

This claim by the English poet has a bearing on Alzheimer's. All humans carry three variations of the Apo E gene, handed down from their parents. One variation has been linked to a high risk of developing Alzheimer's. A study, based on autopsies, found that out of sixty-seven people who carried the Apo E-4 gene, forty-three had been diagnosed with Alzheimer's. Studies of the impact of what your parents fill you up with have on Alzheimer's remain inconclusive. The shudder of fear that passes through a family when a member is diagnosed with dementia originates with the question, Will I be next?

There is nothing you can do about your genes. But a better understanding of the culture in which you grew up and in which you are living can help in dealing with dementia. Culture has been defined in many ways, but can be summarized as "the way we do things around here."

The England in which Pat and I grew up shaped our characters, values, beliefs and the way we saw ourselves. Family background can have a marked effect on how you cope with dementia.

Pat was the eldest of three sisters. I had one older brother who chose a career in health administration and lived a life of undiluted happiness, as he put it, with a wife who never sought to be anything but his companion and a homemaker. Annette, Pat's youngest sister, energetic, vibrant, became a hairdresser, married an Italian doctor and left him for an American professor. Marie, Pat's other sister, loved working on the land and with animals. She was one of the last to be recruited by the Women's Land Army.

Neither Pat nor I came from families with much interest in the arts and culture. Yet we both appreciated good music, especially opera, the theatre, art and literature, although our tastes differed. Pat sympathized with Madame Bovary; I thought she was a dumb broad. I loved *The Iliad* and *The Odyssey*, the first Penguin Classics. Pat had absolutely no interest in Homer and ancient history, which fascinated me.

Was our interest in the arts and the stimulus it gave us a way of escaping from the drab worlds in which we grew up?

Our parents had very different paths through life.

Born in Liverpool in 1886, my father joined the Liverpool Scottish (The King's Regiment), a territorial unit, in 1912.

Tall, well built, he would have looked a fine figure in his kilt and bonnet. The Liverpool Scottish landed in France on November 1, 1914. By December 25, only sixty-five members of the battalion remained in the line; the rest had succumbed to enemy fire or illness.

On June 16, 1915, my father took part in a charge against the enemy lines at Hooge on the Western Front. In this minor action, two-thirds of the Liverpool Scottish, four hundred officers and men, died or were wounded.

My father, slightly wounded, returned to England. A crack shot, he became a musketry instructor. In 1917, he volunteered to join the King's African Rifles and spent the rest of the war chasing Germans and *askaris* (African soldiers) through Tanganyika and Mozambique. Here he caught malaria that stayed with him for the rest of his life.

Dad turned down offers to serve in the Palestine Police and to work on orange farms in South Africa, returning home to be with his mother. Mum was in Liverpool, visiting a relative, when they met. The daughter of a cottar (a farm labourer), she went out to work as a seamstress at an early age. The attraction between my parents appears to have been instantaneous; I sensed, rather than saw, the passion that infused their relationship.

Dad told Mum that he had been "a bit of a lad" — a euphemism for what I gather was a rather riotous life — before they married. She told him she cared nought for his past; they should think only of their future together.

Apparently, my mother and Dad's did not get on very well. Forced to choose between them, he took every penny he possessed, bought a house and severed all connection with his family. My brother arrived in 1926, before the rupture. I came along three years later, after it. Mum's life must have been a lonely one, brought up with five sisters and three brothers in a tightly knit rural family with an extensive kin network. Our family in Liverpool was a very nuclear one.

Returning to "a land fit for heroes," Dad found a job as a left-luggage (baggage) attendant at Central Station. Before lockers appeared, this involved working three shifts, round the clock, with one Sunday off every three weeks. Dad loathed the job, but it meant we had food on the table, a roof over our heads and stayed out of debt.

Pat and I contributed equal amounts to the household budget, but I always saw myself as the main wage earner responsible for my family's needs.

During the blitzes, Dad cycled to work, sometimes shaking with malaria, to relieve his mates. He had no love for the railway company, but knew how important it was for the workers to get back to their families. I learned a sense of responsibility from Dad, an understanding that your first loyalty was to your fellow humans, not to institutions. Whatever happens, you don't let your mates down. Returning from work at night, Dad helped to put out incendiary bombs and throw burning furniture out of houses.

When war broke out in September 1939, my brother was evacuated with his school to Anglesey and I went to stay with my mother's sisters, my maiden aunts, in the village of Oldmeldrum. Mum would never have thought of leaving my father and moving back there. In 1940, my brother and I returned to Liverpool. We had lived as a family and decided, if necessary, to die as one.

Dad's life showed what could happen to a highly able and intelligent person who put security for his family above risk, opportunity and adventure. He died a few years after retiring from his job, having found nothing to do once he stopped work.

Mum, the only one of six sisters to marry, had the traditional Scottish attitude to education, seeing it as a way to get ahead — wherever that was. Her ideas influenced my father, who told me that if I wanted to go to university, he would find the money for me, somehow. Fortunately, I won a scholarship and received an ex-serviceman's grant when I left the Royal Air Force. Mum gave me a mantra that guided my life: "We only go through this life once, so we should do all the good we can for others while we are here."

My brother inherited my parents' good looks. I did not. From time to time, Mum would tell me, "You're afa [awful] ugly." She was astonished when I told her how much I resented this and how it crippled my relationships with women. Although she didn't think much of my face, Mum took great pride in my physique, asking me to strip to the waist to show it to visitors.

I was a late-born child. Mum was thirty-eight when I arrived; Dad was five years older. Our parents did not lavish affection on my brother and I — no hugs, kisses or expressions of affection. But we knew they cared about us, ensured that we were well clothed, fed and housed. Our parents never stopped us doing what we wanted to do; I remember the anguish in my father's eyes as I boarded the train on the first step of my journey to Canada.

When I was about seven or eight, I contracted amebic dysentery, no mean feat in a temperate clime. Liverpool, a port city, had an excellent university department of tropical medicine so the disease was quickly identified and treated. I had lots of diarrhea and messed my hospital bed. A nurse sneered at me, "You're a dirty little thing, aren't you?" I reported this to my father, who went ballistic, stormed into the office of the hospital director and told him, "No one talks to my child like that!"

From this incident, I learned to confront authority on behalf of those being abused. And that if you want to change the music, you must talk to the organ grinder, not to the monkey — that the quest for decency and justice has to begin by telling those at the top of institutions what is happening in the ranks below them. I spent seven or eight weeks in an isolation hospital without seeing my parents. This contributed to my solitary nature.

I learned about Pat's curious family history in bits and pieces. Her parents had not given her the same level of security and stability that mine had. Her mother, Rosamond, born in 1903, came from a family that had lost its main source of income and lived a peripatetic life. George Henry Atkinson, the father, a well-built man with a bushy moustache and a twinkle in his eye, came from a well-heeled background. As a wedding present, his parents gave the couple the Swan Inn in East Ilsley. It flourished until a nearby army base and racing stables, which provided much of the pub's business, moved elsewhere. George, an ardent self-improver, became a perambulating electrician, wiring hotels and large houses. The family moved from High Wycombe to Ross-on-Wye to Torquay, as George found and lost jobs.

Pat's mother recalled an ill-matched couple: "My mother loved life and gaiety, my father loved the country; he had a lathe on which he spent many hours... I remember him as an electrical engineer on large estates, far from civilization."

In the days before electricity came from the grid, big houses had their own generators, which George kept humming. A freethinker, he often quarreled with the owners of the houses. When he was fired, or quit, the family moved to his next job.

Rosamond wrote, "Being the youngest, more time was spent with him, in the Engine House, and he was always trying to explain how, in the future, the atom would be split…and it would be possible to lunch in London and have dinner in New York, the same day. He taught me shorthand at eleven years old and instead of play, it always seemed as if I was transcribing long, uninteresting items from *The Times* or its equivalent."

Did Pat acquire a self-improvement, lifelong learning gene from George? She certainly lived as if she had.

From Rosamond's account, the Atkinsons appear to have been generous and improvident. When the mother and the children — three daughters and a son — arrived at Hazlemere on one move, they expected to be met by George. He was nowhere to be seen. Mrs. Atkinson had spent all her money in Rugby, buying cocoa and cakes for soldiers, and had nothing left to pay for a hotel room. A kindly couple covered the cost of it.

The family lost a daughter in infancy. The son, Harold, enlisted in the army, although he was underage. Sent to France, wounded and invalided out, he volunteered for service in the Middle East. Harold died in battle near Gaza and is buried in the war cemetery there.

One daughter, Dorothy, married a Canadian soldier, moved to Canada, divorced him and returned to England. Gladys, Rosamond's other sister, served in the military in Rugby Camp in 1918. She fell on the ice, dislocated her hip and spent a year in hospital. Developing Munchausen syndrome, she took up a career as a professional invalid, lying in bed, much admired by all for her bravery and stoicism.

Pat's mother became the strong one in the family, running the house, caring for her aging parents "who were getting worn out" and looking after Aunty Glad. A photo shows the family clustered around her as she sits, relaxed, in a wheelchair. Pat stands beside it, hugging her teddy bear.

Rosamond married Frank Wicks around the age of twenty-five. A wedding photo shows both sets of parents with the newlywed couple. Frank's father, a teacher, tall, good looking, wears a business suit; Mr. Atkinson and the groom are in morning dress. The three women, all elegantly dressed, carry enormous bouquets of flowers. The wedding, as the British say, must have cost a few bob, for it looks like a very posh affair.

Rosamond, a very beautiful, strong-minded woman, had three beautiful daughters. When I went with them to the opera in Rome, all eyes, male and female, swiveled in their direction as we walked down the aisle. They certainly were not looking at me!

Pat's mother wrote of Pat, "She was the most beautiful baby — and so brave when she had paralysis after diphtheria; she never gave up... In a way she was so different — but not really difficult. She was so honest, with such willpower..."

A photo shows Patricia Ann about the age of two. She looks very determined, staring at the camera somewhat resentfully.

In *Musicophilia*, Oliver Sacks writes, "It seems certain... that in the first two years of life...deep emotional memories and associations are...being made in the limbic system and other regions of the brain... These emotional memories may determine one's behaviour for a lifetime."

Unlike me, Pat grew up in an extended family. Yet, like me, she had a solitary nature. Looking at her photo, which hangs in our home, I wonder what emotional memories were already fixed in the mind of this beautiful two-year-old that gave her such a look of stubbornness and defiance. The few photos I have of Pat with her mother and sisters show the children well and neatly dressed and obviously well nurtured.

For reasons I never fathomed, and about which she never spoke, Pat harboured deep-seated anger against her mother; she was furious when Rosamond announced she was coming to our wedding. Pat's sister Marie believed that the antagonism arose between them because "they were very much alike." Determined, strong-minded, both had made their own way through life.

I picked up Pat's feelings about her mother and treated her rather unkindly when she visited us, developing a convenient headache to retire from her presence. As I came to know her better, I saw in her many admirable qualities. She had been the anchor of the family, caring for parents and her children. Her mother-in-law, a snob, looked down on her, believing her son had married beneath his station. An intelligent, able woman, Rosamond had made a life for herself outside marriage, becoming involved in the St. John's Ambulance and rising to a senior rank in it.

Pat reconciled with her mother before she died. She designed a front entrance for our unit in Thorndean featuring stained glass (plastic actually) side windows with large roses, in memory of her mother.

When last I saw Rosamond, she asked me for advice on keeping her assets out of the hands of her husband, Frank. By this time, they had separated and Frank had another woman — her name never mentioned — in his life. Although Pat was close to her father, she spoke little about him and he did not make a strong impression on me. Frank had a furtive, sideways-glancing look as if forever seeking for the door marked Exit. He spent his working life with the telephone section of the post office after being hired for his skill as a football player: the Brighton office needed one for its team.

Like my father, Frank spent his entire life in one job. But he showed some enterprise when he and a friend ran a book at a local racetrack. When they discovered they did not have enough money to cover the bets, the partners decamped before the punters arrived for their payouts.

Frank died in 1983, apparently suffering from dementia. Did he pass on the rogue gene of it to Pat? Another mystery about her, among so many others.

Small events in childhood, youth and adolescence, of which we recall little, if anything, can have major influences in later life. George Mackay Brown, the Orcadian writer, observed, "No man is an island, and all that we ever say or think or do — however seemingly unremarkable — may yet set the whole web of existence trembling and affect the living and the dead and the unborn."

Pat and I leapt from the web of our families and began to weave our separate webs and then a joint one that enmeshed us and others. Coming from different cultural and family backgrounds, we proved surprisingly compatible. We both had a great curiosity about the world and wanted to keep on learning about its ways. I had an optimistic, cheerful view of life, although I went through periods of depression after we married. Pat's seriousness, reflected in "the sorrows of her changing face," attracted me, and I tried to alleviate it.

We had no great and ambitious goals as we set out on our life together — no dreams of success. We had a strong sense of the need to be of service to others — without making nuisances of ourselves.

We did not want to follow in the footsteps of our fathers. We wanted interesting and challenging jobs and the chance to travel. And we found them — and places we loved to visit.

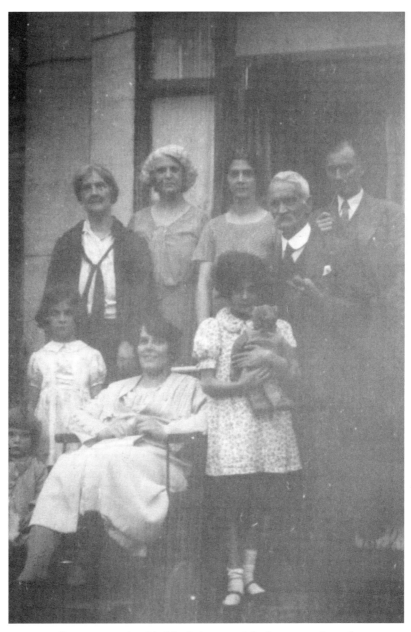

Pat, aged seven, with "Teddy." Auntie Glad is seated in the wheelchair with Pat's sisters to the left, and her parents and grandparents behind.

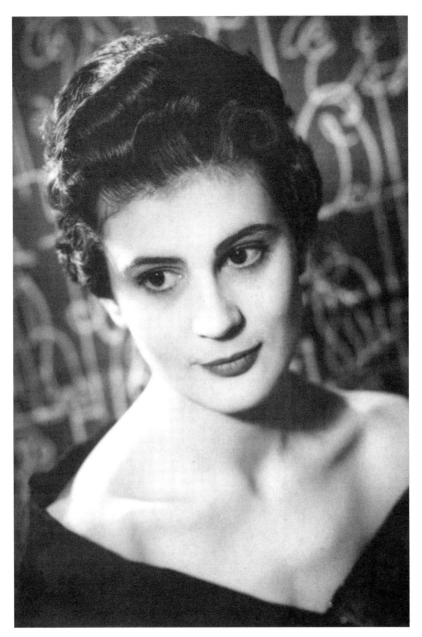

Pat, Montreal, 1957.

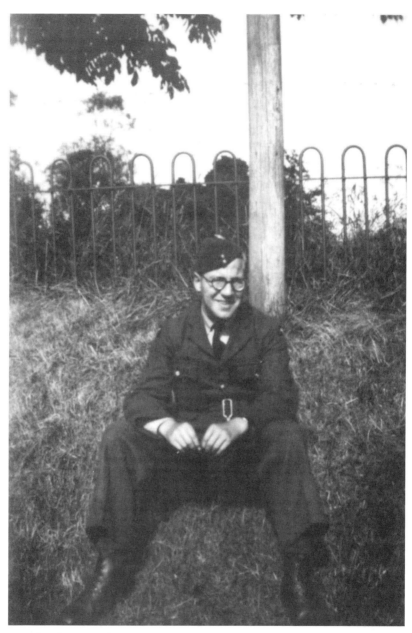

Jim, in the Royal Air Force, somewhere in Wiltshire, 1947.

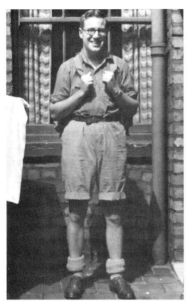

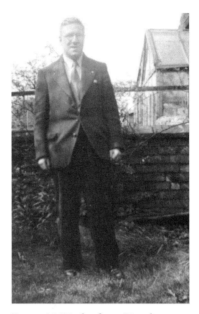

In the yard at Jim's Liverpool home after hitch-hiking across North Africa, 1950.

June 1950, before Jim leaves England.

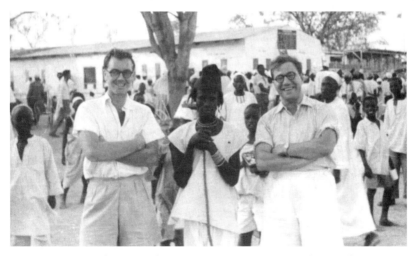

Brian Sagar and Jim at the Kano Races, 1950, with a Fulani herdsman. The herdsman said he wanted to be in the photograph, though he does not seem happy about it.

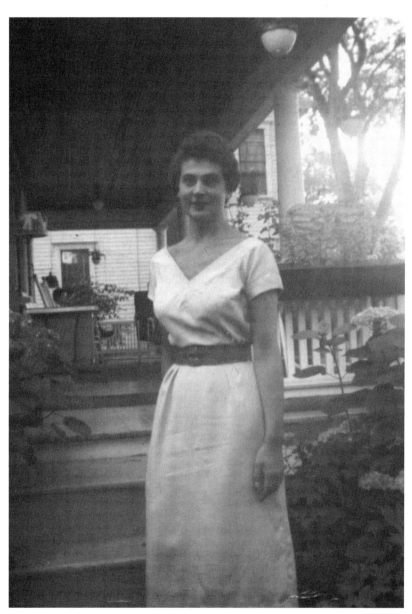

Pat in Montreal, 1955.

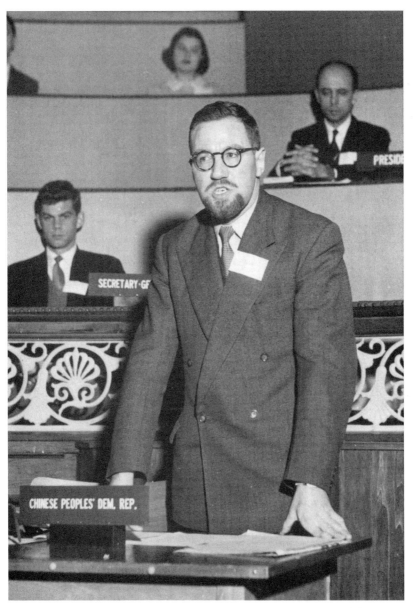

Jim representing the Chinese Peoples' Democratic Republic at
a mock United Nations, McGill University, 1956. When he lost
a vote, he did what the Chinese delegation would have done —
walked out of the session!

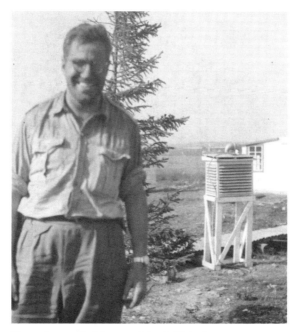

Jim after a field trip, McGill Subarctic
Research Laboratory, July 1956.

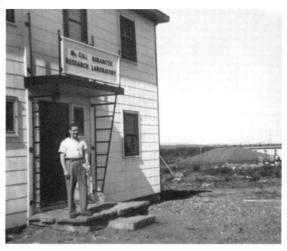

At the entrance to the lab, setting out to
measure the height of a cloud.

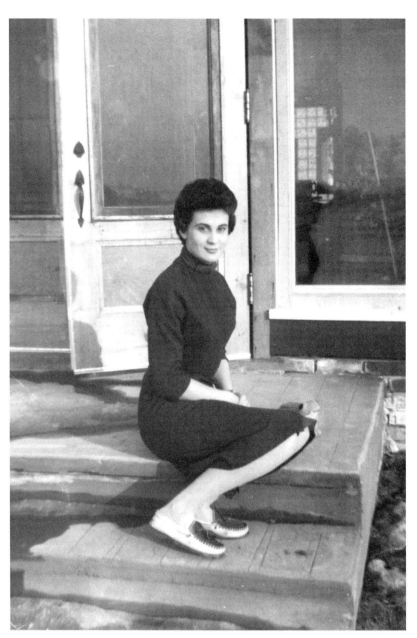

Pat at Varennes, 1955.

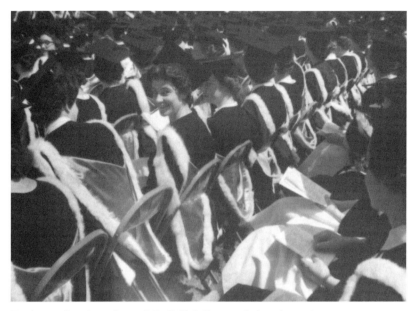

Pat's graduation from McGill Library School, 1959.

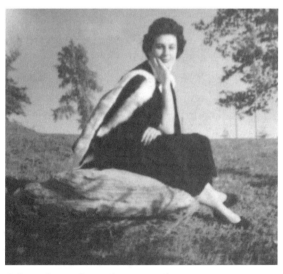

A less formal graduation photo, 1959.

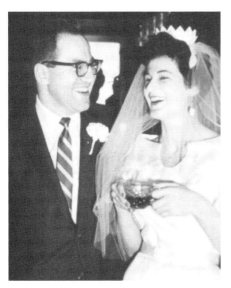 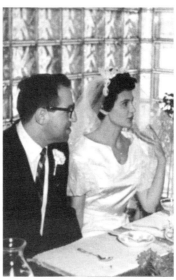

Wedding Day, December 12, 1959.

Jim and Pat at their wedding reception.

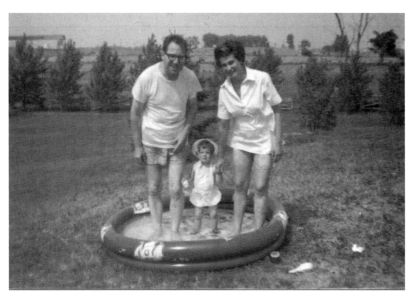

Jim and Pat with daughter Annette in 1962, near Varennes at a farm managed by Pat's sister Marie.

Chapter Four
Work, Travel, Study

All that matters is love and work.

Sigmund Freud

Pat and I had lots of love in our married life.

After moving to Halifax in 1973, we had trouble finding work. Pat, as a professional librarian, always had a better chance of finding a good job than did I. When we married, I still had not decided what I wanted to do when I grew up. Canadian employers, a conservative lot, looked over my resume: radio fitter, trader in Africa, glacial meteorologist, cartographer, advertising copywriter. I left out opera super, grouse beater, toy salesperson, farm labourer and truck driver's assistant to avoid confusing the interviewer further. A recruiter for a large corporation told me, "If we find anything unusual to do, we'll contact you." These days, of course, I would be seen to have high social, economic and geographical mobility, desirable characteristics in an employee.

Becoming Canadian

Pat and I carried with us to Canada a strong work ethic.

You did your best for those who hired you, no matter how lowly or unrewarding the work or how much you received for it.

As newcomers to Canada, we had to learn about the way things were done here and adapt to them as best we could. During our time together, the country moved slowly from under the influence of Britain and acquired beliefs, values and practices from the United States. Canada borrowed the concept of the Welfare State from Britain and the tradition of fumbling through and pragmatism. Through the 1960s and up to the present, the American faith in the so-called free market, professionalism and the belief that every problem has an instant solution dominated thought in Canada. Understatement and modesty, key aspects of the British character, gave way to hype, naiveté, aggressiveness, the worship of celebrity and other unappealing parts of American culture.

Coming from the restricted world of working-class England, Pat and I saw Canada as a land of promise. It lacked the over exuberance, energy and individualism of the United States and the ant-like conformity so marked in European nations. We liked the absence of a well-defined national identity in Canada, having suffered from an excess of it in Britain, the "Land of Hope and Glory," with the plea that "God who made us mighty/ Make us mightier yet."

Canada, to us, resembled Shaw's definition of marriage, which he claimed combined "the maximum of temptation with the maximum of opportunity." When Pat graduated from library school she found plenty of employers eager to hire her and her classmates.

I liked Alden Nowlan's vision of Canada as less like a traditional nation-state than as "magnificent raw material" for creating one: "Perhaps the question is not who we are, but 'what are we going to make of ourselves?'"

That question intrigued Pat and I at the personal level as we set out to find opportunities for individual and joint development and for ways we could aid the growth of a new nation and a new society. I believe that many immigrants feel this way about Canada. We were not interested simply in bettering ourselves. We also sought to contribute whatever skills, abilities and experiences we had acquired to others. We had made a choice to leave an established way of life, family and friends, to make a new one for ourselves, to write a new narrative. We wanted to participate in the making of a new kind of country, one free of the ills and limitations of the one in which we grew up.

An encounter I had while directing a research project in Basse-Ville, Ottawa's Lower Town, in 1966 gave me some insights into the beliefs and values of Canadians. The city planned to drive a highway through the area without informing and involving local residents. I joined a committee to coordinate (a euphemism for control) activities in this working-class part of Ottawa. At a meeting, a social worker claimed that when poor people moved into public housing in Britain they kept coal in their bathtubs. I corrected her: "They gave poor people coal scuttles and they insisted on taking baths in them." I was "deselected" from the committee by not being informed of meetings. My subversive sense of humour brought into question the parochialism, middle-class morality and concern for propriety of many professionals in Canada.

We had a glimpse of how middle-class Canadians lived during a vacation in Northern Ontario. Pat decided we should have a week at a rural retreat with activities for our daughters. At the resort on Lake Rosseau, that programme consisted of two bored teenagers handing out crayons and pages ripped from colouring books. Annette and Fiona did not take kindly to this and were labeled troublemakers. Each evening the bouncy recreation director would bounce up to our table and invite us to take part in the next day's activities. We politely refused his offer. The people in the next cabin invited us in "for a drink." We joined a group of Torontonians whose holiday consisted of drinking as much booze as possible in as short a time as possible. Maybe living in Toronto in those days did that to you. We declined further invitations for drinks. Fortunately, a railway strike loomed and we escaped from the resort a day or two early.

Pat and I delighted in the egalitarianism and lack of class-consciousness we encountered in Canada and the general friendliness and politeness of the people we met. They did appear somewhat reclusive, disinclined to confront arbitrary authority and far too dependent on government to solve their problems. Doing the research for my books on Canadian military history, I saw how this country's soldiers, sailors and airmen, given the toughest tasks, acquited themselves with courage and dedication. A poet, I think it was E. J. Pratt, described Canadians as "the stunted strong." A famous definition of them is "someone who apologizes when someone stands on their foot."

After we acquired our own house in Ottawa in 1965, we joined the middle class. But we never fitted into it or had any desire to do so. In Canada, we found, you could live your life as an individual and work with others on ventures of mutual interest. From time to time we joined middle-class causes. I served as chair of the Ottawa chapter of the Canadian Campaign for Nuclear Disarmament. Pat became a member of The Voice of Women and lobbied for peace.

We tired of trying to solve all the problems of Canada and the world. Pat had much more satisfaction serving meals to poor kids in the North End of Halifax, or putting together a book on heritage homes, than from sitting on committees dedicated to eradicating some real or imagined evil.

We remained "unCanadian" in many ways.

Neither of us participated in or watched sports, although I had been captain of the McGill judo team. We thought hockey brutal, football and baseball boring. We never barbecued anything on our back porch or had the urge to come close to nature by acquiring a cottage in the country, especially as mosquitoes took a special delight in feasting on Pat.

Lacking a car, we walked a lot. Claims have been made that exercise, including walking, can delay Alzheimer's and I wonder if this was the case with Pat. The lack of a car meant we spent a lot of time at home. Pat turned our homes into comfortable, restful and welcoming places. This had a considerable impact on how we dealt with her dementia. Pat felt safe in our familiar, well-loved condo in a beautiful old building.

We realized soon after we married that ours would not be a conventional marriage with Pat staying at home while I held a steady job. She certainly did not marry me for money or for my career prospects, for they were very uncertain. I had reached my level of competence in meteorology and would need more math and physics to advance in this field. I certainly did not want to spend months in the Arctic, away from Pat, especially as she was pregnant with Annette, our first daughter.

In 1960, Geoff Hattersley-Smith, leader of Operation Hazen, arranged a six-month contract with the Defence Research Board, and we moved from Montreal to an apartment in Riverview (now Vanier City) a suburb of Ottawa, where I edited reports and wrote technical papers. I also searched, desperately, for work to support my new family.

In the fall of 1960, I found a job as a community planner with the Department of Northern Affairs. Six weeks after Annette was born, I flew to Whitehorse to do a study of the squatters who lived on the fringes of the Yukon's capital. As the territory developed, became bureaucratized and its residents more "respectable," the squatters, a holdover from the boom days and a response to the uncertainty of life in a marginal area of Canada, were seen as a problem, a blight on the cityscape. Stereotyped as people who did not pay city taxes and "guys shacked up with Indian women," these undesirables on Whiskey Flats and Moccasin Flats had to go.

I spent several weeks interviewing hundreds of squatters and those involved with them and was always treated with great courtesy and respect. I soon discovered that squatters were not a breed apart but lived pretty much like other Yukoners and formed a vital part of the city's economy.

Back in Ottawa, I wrote my report, which was well received. Fancies about the squatters had been replaced by facts.

Governments live on paperwork, on reports, memos, policy papers that pin down problems and clarify options.

My skill in writing reports ensured my future in the federal civil service. I was more interested in solving problems than in writing about them.

Our second daughter, Fiona, was born in 1962.

I always wanted Pat to have a career of her own. Ahead of her time, she became a working mother after we arranged for care for our daughters. They were proud their mum had a job. Pat worked as an editor with the Canadian Periodical Index. As a community planner, I visited Inuvik, Frobisher Bay (now Iqaluit), Thompson, Uranium City and Dawson City on specific assignments or to prepare community studies.

In 1963, I joined the Northern Coordination and Research Centre, part of the office of the deputy minister, and focused my research on the Yukon. This marginal part of Canada, where residents adapted in different ways to the uncertainty of the environment and the economy, intrigued me. Visits to the territory initiated a lifelong interest in social and economic development on the edges of industrialized countries.

Pat accepted my need to follow my interests wherever they led and to have a life in which she did not participate, no matter how close we became. In the summers of 1963 and 1964, which I spent in the Yukon, Pat took our daughters to Italy, where her sister lived, and to Scotland. Pat's fascination with the land of the haggis and heather would influence our lives in later years.

In the fall of 1964, I took educational leave from the government and enrolled in the Ph.D. programme in geography at the University of British Columbia. Graduate accommodation consisted of old army shacks through whose paper-thin walls the winter wind whistled relentlessly. If you drove a nail into a wall, your next-door neighbour could hang a picture on it. We acquired some rudimentary bits of furniture, living in squalor while enjoying a rich community life with other graduates with whom we had lively discussions.

I suffered from role shock and institution shock.

The university had just launched the doctoral programme, and it soon became obvious to me that those running it had no idea how to treat mature students. As a middle level civil servant, I had a responsible job and the resources I needed to do it. Graduate students in geography were treated like high school students. I marvel now at the way Pat and the kids put up with me as I teetered on the brink of madness. I shouted, cursed, banged my fists on the walls of our shack. Pat suggested I see the campus doctor. He advised me to take her out more often. This encounter made me skeptical about the ability of doctors to appreciate and understand the context of the lives of patients and influenced how I cared for Pat.

My graduate career ended with a disastrous oral exam. I had been involved in research for ten years, published scientific papers and done other academic things. Oral exams, however, are not directed at letting you tell others what you know. They aim to humiliate you by finding out what you don't know. I did not take kindly to this and flunked the oral. What I learned at UBC about the treatment of students influenced the way I dealt with them when I became a professor at another university eight months later.

I felt strangely relieved at being ejected from the university. Pat and I decided the family would spend the summer of 1965 in Whitehorse while I continued my research. In contrast to our living quarters on the UBC campus, we occupied a large, fully furnished house on the old army base of Camp Takhini. We met the territorial librarian who was about to go on leave and asked Pat, as the only other professional librarian in the city, to take her place while she was away. Yukoners proved very hospitable and Pat put on dinner parties for some we met.

We decided to buy a house on our return to Ottawa. Pat found a splendid one in the Glebe, and it became a restful place for us, the kids and our visitors.

In 1965, Ottawa had the ambiance of a small town. While in the downtown one day, I saw Prime Minister Lester Pearson in earnest conversation with Maurice Strong, one of Canada's power elite. Passing the Parliament Buildings, I caught a glimpse of Pierre Elliott Trudeau, Pearson's successor, walking alone from the East Block to the Centre Block.

In 1966, I was seconded to the commission on the government of the Northwest Territories (the Carrothers Commission) to survey social science research there. As I finished this assignment, I had a choice of futures. As Yogi Berra put it, "When you come to a fork in the road, take it."

I was offered the position of research director on the War on Poverty in the Privy Council Office, the centre of power in Canada. I had been teaching community development at the University of Ottawa, which was run by the Oblates of Mary Immaculate, a missionary order. To secure government grants, it split into a secular body, the University of Ottawa, and a religious one, Université St. Paul. Father Champagne, head of its Institute of Missiology, invited me to teach there and to serve as assistant director of the Canadian Research Centre for Anthropology.

I accepted his offer and it proved to be the right choice.

Growing up in Liverpool, I had been taught that if I

touched a Catholic, I would break out in a rash. At St. Paul, I had freedom to follow my research interests on marginal places and people while teaching nuns, priests and laypeople.

Had I joined the Privy Council Office, I would have been restrained and constrained by bureaucratic limits on what I could and could not do. As in the United States, the poor lost the war on poverty and the agencies set up to run it vanished into limbo.

I had a glimpse of what our married life might have been like had I become a senior government official. While I was learning French, the wife of a senior official asked the instructor, "What's the difference between *vous* and *tu* when you address someone?" He explained that the first was used in formal interactions, the second implied warmth, intimacy, affection. "You would not hear much of that in our home," the woman sadly replied.

I know that Pat would have supported me had I joined the Privy Council Office and played the role ascribed to her. We avoided this fate and remained in a tu/toi relationship to the end of her days.

After I joined Université St. Paul, Pat freelanced as an editor. Through our home on Second Avenue passed anthropologists, geographers, sociologists, Inuit, members of the First Nations, African-Americans, graduate students from the United States, British professors, delinquent youth and radicals from Canada and elsewhere in the world. Some stayed with us, others enjoyed Pat's excellent meals.

Annette and Fiona grew up colour blind, learning the first law of hospitality: "Guests come first." We raised them in a somewhat absent-minded way, taking care of their needs, doing all we could to ensure their safety, health and happiness, giving them plenty of love, letting them find their own way through the world, with our backing and support, taking them with us on our travels.

Scotland

We both longed to spend time in Scotland. Pat had become intrigued with its history, and I wanted to look at life in the Highlands and Islands. In the summer of 1968, we rented a cottar house, like the one in which my mother was born, in Croy, a small village near Inverness. This proved to be a golden time for us as I researched the region and joined Pat and the kids on country rambles, visiting castles and learning about their history. The characters that interest people tell you a lot about them.

Pat stumbled on the story of Alexander Stewart, Earl of Mar, "a leader of broken men and the terror of the countryside" according to one historian, "a most personable scoundrel" in the words of another. Born the bastard son of the Earl of Buchan, "The Wolf of Badenoch," in 1375, Stewart laid siege to Kildrummy Castle as part of his strategy to wed its owner, the Countess of Mar, to secure an earldom. We visited this place, and Lochindorb Castle where Stewart was born, a grim ruin on an island surrounded by bare land once covered by the Caledonian Forest.

The wild Highlander became leader of an army of Lowlanders defending Aberdeen against an attack by Donald, Lord of the Isles and his six thousand followers. They met on July 24, 1411, at Harlaw, a few kilometres from my mother's village. Hundreds died on that day with neither side claiming victory. The Highlanders retreated and Stewart gained credit for saving Aberdeen. A sandstone obelisk amid fields of golden grain marks this savage encounter.

We located a beheaded statue of the earl in a church-yard behind the Inverness telephone exchange. Pat thought about writing a novel about him. Instead, she published an article in the October 1970 issue of the *Northern Counties Magazine*. Headed "In Search of the Earl of Mar," it ended, "On the anniversary of his death [August 1, 1345 or 1346] we paid our tribute to Alexander Stewart. We walked down to Greyfriars Churchyard, untied the wire holding the gates together and squeaked one open. At the foot of the Earl of Mar's effigy we placed three red roses and quietly walked away."

Did Pat see something of this wild man in me? Or was she simply fascinated by someone who managed to bridge the gap between the two worlds of Scotland: the settled life in Aberdeen and the random brutality of the country's untamed interior?

We had many magical moments in Scotland. Walking back to Croy one evening, we passed a poultry barn where caged birds dropped their eggs onto an endless belt. Opposite lay a patch of untamed heath and sand where we saw the rabbits dancing. They chased each other, flipped into the air, threw themselves around in wild confusion, romped about, dashed in and out of burrows. We stood, transfixed, as twilight descended, watching these strange antics, which may have been mating rituals or simply sheer exuberance. They made a striking contrast to the regimented and restricted lives of the hens on the other side of the road.

We had another wonderful experience during a summer on Mull, one of the Inner Hebrides islands. In 1970, we rented a large, drafty house near Dervaig on the north coast.

Locals told us that the weather had been beautiful before we arrived, and the day of our departure proved clear and sunny. In between those times, it rained and rained and rained as only it can in western Scotland. Each day we would don rain gear and head for Dervaig to buy groceries. On rare sunny days we climbed nearby hills and marveled at the beauty of the rugged landscape. And we visited a sheep farm to see the animals being clipped and dipped.

The sacred island of Iona, once the centre of Celtic Christianity, lies off the southwest tip of Mull and we determined to visit it. Suitably dressed to ward off the ever-present rain, we reached Fionnphort and boarded the boat for Iona. Here we had another magical moment as we set off for the island. We knew no one else on board. A great peace settled upon us, a sudden sense of tranquility and community with everyone else on the boat. We smiled at each other, no longer strangers, recognizing that each of us had embarked on a pilgrimage, not merely a boat journey. This sense of instant community lasted until the boat docked at Iona and we went our separate ways, spiritually refreshed.

I had a five-year contract with the university, drawn up by myself, that would last until the fall of 1971. On our return from Scotland, I discovered that my boss, Father Jean Trudeau, had quit the priesthood and his job. Jean had let me run the Canadian Research Centre for Anthropology in my own way. I directed studies of unemployed youth in Ottawa and squatting in Canada, taught community development and ran the centre's publications programme, with Pat as editor. Jean had been a buffer between me and the university administrators, with whom I had limited contact. These priests would now directly supervise what I did. I completed reports on the research projects and handed in my resignation.

We had an interesting life in Ottawa. I enjoyed teaching mature students — and learning from them. I continued my research on community development, helping to organize a conference on it at the University of Missouri. I visited the University of Alaska several times, took part in Glenn Gould's radio programme and film "The Idea of North" and served on a panel at Expo '67 with the eccentric genius Buckminster Fuller; his colleague the futurist John McHale; Moshe Safdie, designer of Habitat; Ralph Erskine, a Swedish-based British architect who designed northern communities; and economics professor George Rogers from the University of Alaska. During a lunch together, I turned to Bucky Fuller, who was sitting next to me, and said, "I'm always expecting someone to tap me on the shoulder in places like this and say, 'We know about you — out!'" Bucky laughed and replied, "I feel the same way."

Pat ran her own business in Ottawa as an editor, doing various "jobbies" as she called them and selling stories to children's magazines.

Both of us could have joined the expanding civil service and retired on pension, but neither of us wanted a life of routine in an office. We felt we were in a rut and sought new challenges. And we certainly found them!

Antigonish

While at St. Paul, I had been contacted by a representative of the Ford Foundation. It was running a programme in Canada that gave potential leaders $15,000 to develop their abilities in any way they wanted. I pointed out to the Ford man that Canada had a culture of institutions, not of individualism as prevailed in the United States. I offered to attach the people he selected for the leadership programme to the Canadian Research Centre for Anthropology as research associates to give them an institutional identity. Wayne Patterson, an African-Canadian (a term not used at the time) from Saint John, took up my offer and we became friends.

Pat and I decided that since we enjoyed life in Old Scotland, I would seek a job in New Scotland, Nova Scotia. Wayne met us in Fredericton and drove us around the province. We had an odd experience entering a restaurant in a small town. People stared at us. A white couple and a black man? What's going on here? I was offered a two-year contract to teach community development at Coady International Institute at St. Francis Xavier University in Antigonish.

I took it. We returned to Ottawa to sell our house. Pat bought a large six-bedroom one in Greenwold, just outside the town limits. We had an interesting introduction to life in rural Nova Scotia. The family travelled by train to Antigonish, dumped our luggage at the station and headed into town for breakfast. On our return, we saw a young man standing at the roadside with what looked like one of our bags. He claimed it was his. Pat knelt down, zipped it open, pulled out several sanitary napkins and asked him, "Do you use many of these?" He fled.

Pat had a *Wind in the Willows* view of rural life, which I did not share. Ever the romantic, she fell in love with Antigonish with its broad main street, white churches and sense of always afternoon. Opportunities for her to use her skills were few, so Pat decided to enjoy life in the country with our two daughters. We lived in the county, so they were bussed to a school on the highway. Seasoned travellers, they spoke about their experiences in class. Other students, some of whom had not even been to Halifax, resented this and showed their displeasure. Our daughters learned to keep their mouths shut.

We decided to join the Antigonish Highland Society.

I qualified because my mother was Scottish. Pat and I stood with other inductees as we gave our tribal affiliations: Maclean! MacDonald! McLaren! Lotz! McVitie! McBain!

We never received invitations to any of the society's meetings.

We took the kids on rural rambles on the weekends and drove to Cheticamp with friends. Pat invited the Coady students in batches to meals in our home. But we made few friends in this tightly knit community. And we became increasingly aware of undertones of racism.

Pat volunteered to work with Girl Guides and Cubs and was disturbed when she encountered racism when black members came to Antigonish from the community of Lincolnville. Annette invited a black friend to her birthday party. Later, she came to Pat, puzzled. A white friend of hers had asked her, "Does your mother know the girl you invited is black?" Why had she asked this question? Annette was completely baffled.

We soon realized we were not small-town rural people.

Pat and I did research for our book on Cape Breton, not very amicably as we argued over who would write which parts of it. In her diary on January 1, 1972, Pat wrote, "I wish I were earning some money, but the opportunities around here are severely limited." She added, "I have found the entire holiday season rather a lonely one, despite having Coady students over for Christmas Day and Boxing Day. The old saying that small towns are friendly simply is not true, except in a very superficial way. However, living in a small community is a valuable experience — heck! it has to be something."

Seeking a challenge, Pat enrolled in the master's degree programme in Celtic Studies at St. Francis Xavier University. She enjoyed the courses, began to learn Gaelic, wrote her thesis on Scottish societies in Nova Scotia (*Scots in Groups*) and received her degree in 1975.

The university did not renew my contract in 1973, so we decided to move to Halifax and see if we could make a living there. Like many others in her class, Pat had read about the wonders of life in exclusive girls' boarding schools from books like *The Fourth Form at St. Camiknicks*. She had not had the experience, but decided Annette should. So we enrolled her in Edgehill School in Windsor and moved to the big city.

Halifax and Thorndean

We had no idea how we would make a living in a city where we had no contacts or friends. We agreed that Pat should look for a job while I freelanced. Pat accepted that I would have difficulty in regular employment after the autonomy I'd enjoyed in government and university. Halifax and Nova Scotia were highly ascriptive parts of Canada; who you knew counted for much more than what you could do.

In 1970, the federal government set up Information Canada to keep citizens aware of its activities. Pat found a term position with the agency. Here again, she was ahead of her time. Librarians, hooked on books, did not realize they were in the information business. Pat, fluently bilingual, took an exam and became head of enquiry officers in the

Halifax office of Information Canada. I seldom dropped into her office, believing that it was essential that Pat have her own identity and place apart from me. She did an excellent job at the short-lived agency.

Judith Ryan, one of Pat's staff, recalled her as being "fair, straightforward and [trusting] in my ability to do my job with minimal supervision." When Judith went freelance, Pat encouraged her and gave her references and contacts.

Pat lost her job at Information Canada when the government abolished it in 1975. As a civil servant, she had to be found a new one and moved over to Consumer and Corporate Affairs as district manager in charge of enquiries. She wrote articles for community newspapers and magazines, did radio broadcasts and organized workshops and activities for young people. Pat accepted a woman on social assistance on a work placement in her office and ensured she was treated with dignity and respect. When a permanent position with the department in Vancouver was posted, Pat and her staff encouraged the woman to apply for it. She won the competition and set off for a new life on the west coast.

In 1979, the department reorganized and Pat was "declared surplus."

And we moved into Thorndean.

On our walks, we'd passed a mansion on Inglis Street in the South End area of Halifax. "I would love to live there," said Pat. "It's a cooperative." Thorndean, an elegant Georgian house, had fallen on hard times in the 1960s before the upsurge of interest in heritage buildings. The Rozinskis, he Polish, she Belgian, bought the place and renovated it with the help of sailors from Polish ships. We heard stories of their furtive arrivals and departures in the dark of night. As we learned in maintaining the building, they had more enthusiasm than knowledge when it came to renovation. The Rosinskis created five apartments and decided to sell the building. The tenants wanted to stay in this beautiful house but Nova Scotia, at that time, did not have condominium legislation. They formed a residential shareholders' corporation and bought shares in it based on the size of their units. The building became a condominium in 1984.

One day Pat noticed a small newspaper ad for an apartment.

"That's Thorndean!" she exclaimed. How she knew this I never did discover. She phoned the number in the ad and we rushed over to meet the owners. I recall Pat sitting, hands clasped as if to check her enthusiasm, completely entranced with the high ceilings and spacious rooms of Thorndean. Built in 1834–38, its first owner, James Forman, had been cashier of the Bank of Nova Scotia and a pillar of Halifax society. The house, when built, stood alone in the open countryside.

I could live in a cave, having spent time in the Arctic in tents, and never wanted to own much beyond my clothes and a few books. I always relied on Pat to pick the places where we would live.

We quickly agreed to the owners' price and bought their shares in the corporation. Thorndean proved to be an ideal dwelling place for walkers like us. Point Pleasant Park was within easy walking distance, a supermarket stood nearby. Saint Mary's University lay up the street and the Atlantic School of Theology, which Pat and I attended, about twenty minutes' walk away.

Pat loved Thorndean with all its faults: kitchen taps that froze in winter, water-saturated ceilings that suddenly collapsed, front rooms that leaked in rainstorms, a too-hot stove and a too-cold fridge. Over the years, we corrected many of these problems. Pat had the front room for her study while I took the Regency Room for mine. It overlooked a large garden, to which Pat applied her gardening skills. Our antique furniture fitted well into this old house.

We acquired a cat in our usual, unusual way.

Dino had been abandoned by his owners and picked up by the children of a woman allergic to cats. With her characteristic kindness, Fiona brought it home with her. Dino looked over the place, decided he liked it, settled in and became very fond of Pat. We delighted in Dino's independent streak; he went out every evening and returned each morning. We discovered that he had been popping into a ground-floor unit in the apartment building next door to be fed by its owner. He died in 1991. Pat tried to find a replacement, but Dino had spoiled us for other cats and she did not find one. When Pat was suffering from dementia, a friend tried pet therapy with her, bringing over a kitten. Pat was terrified of it, just one indication of how she changed.

Each year, beginning about 1996, Pat organized an All Broads' Brunch, cooking all the food herself. She did not do this to network or make contacts or to impress her friends. She simply wanted to give them a joyful experience in a beautiful house. All the women she invited had strong personalities; most were involved in writing in some way. Judith Ryan recalled the brunches as resembling "an old-fashioned salon, where [Pat] brought together women of varied pursuits and accomplishments, indicative of her own broad and eclectic interests."

I did not attend the brunches, but was allowed to do the washing-up and to eat the leftovers. I never resented my exclusion, delighting in the way these gatherings enhanced

Pat's life and those of her friends. Pat's initiative in organizing these events illustrated a central feature of our life together. She had to do the things that were important to her on her own, in her way. Though we loved each other deeply, and more and more as the years went by, we recognized that we each had to follow our own interests. Pat had no interest in community development, the field in which I had been immersed since 1960. I had little concern for heritage preservation, which attracted Pat's attention.

After living in Thorndean for a few months, we knew it had always been a happy home. It proved to be an ideal place to care for Pat. Our unit, all on one floor, had no internal stairs that she had to navigate, only a short flight to the front path. The tranquil view over the back garden gave us both solace in difficult times, especially when the sun streamed through the bay windows.

Pat had her dream home.

And she found her dream job.

After leaving government, she became copyeditor of *Atlantic Insight*, a glossy regional magazine. Roma Arsenault, who worked with her, recalled, "We met in 1978, before the launch of *Atlantic Insight*. Pat was elegant, personable and knew so much about so many things. I'd had a couple of jobs in journalism, but I had much to learn and Pat, in her quiet way, taught me a lot about research skills, grammar and life. In the early years, *Atlantic Insight* was a fun, positive place to work, and we were all enthusiastic about helping to produce something good. Pat, Pam [Lutz], and I shared the front room in that lovely house on Coburg Road. We all got along, laughed a lot and worked hard."

Pam Lutz wrote, "[Pat] was a mentor and I learned more about editing from her than any other person before or since." Pat became associate editor, wrote articles for the magazine and served as food editor. She resigned in 1984, on a matter of principle, when new owners confused advertising with editorial copy.

Pat had nothing in mind when she quit the magazine. She had enrolled in the masters of theology studies (MTS) programme at the Atlantic School of Theology (AST) to reconnect with her Anglican roots. Seeking to read the Old and New Testaments in their original languages, she learned Hebrew and Greek; Post-it notes with strange characters on them blossomed on the doors and walls of our home.

One evening, after Pat had left *Atlantic Insight*, we stood in the living room hugging each other. Pat told me that she wanted to attend AST on a full-time basis. By this time I was earning enough money to support us and encouraged Pat to do this. Almost on the same day, I noticed an ad for an editor of *The Southender*, a community newspaper. Pat applied for the position and was hired to run, eventually, two community newspapers with a circulation of about thirty-five thousand. She took courses at AST while editing the newspapers.

At first she worked at the office until two in the morning, pasting down copy and ads. I bought her a computer — which I never learned to use — and she was home in time for tea on the day the paper went to the printers. Pat found columnists who had never written for newspapers, nurturing them and other contributors, ran short stories and turned the paper into a source of information on Halifax.

She also became editor of *The Westender*. She wrote stories on the Jewish community in Halifax, and the Welsh one, on the cathedral ("Why All Saints is topless"), on Third Age Housing and teddy bear mania. Pat did not use the paper as a pulpit but did include religious stories. When rumours circulated that a group of Tibetan Buddhists, who had moved their centre from Boulder, Colorado, were taking over the Halifax development industry, Pat asked me to write a story on them. I also did one on faith healing. As I told people, the paper did not pay much, ten cents a word, but I was allowed to sleep with the editor.

By now our daughters had left home, Annette to join the Canadian Forces, Fiona to take a job with Canadian Tire and rent her first apartment. Both loved rather too well than too wisely, having inherited Pat's kind nature or absorbed it by example. Fiona complained how difficult it was for her to find a suitable mate after seeing how much Pat and I loved each other: "You set such a high standard."

Pat's innocence, one of the many qualities about her that I loved, cost her money. When she became editor of *The Southender*, I suggested she secure a contract with the publisher that contained a condition that she receive six months' severance pay should he sell the paper. She did not do so. In September 1989, she was shocked to discover that the papers had been sold and that she was not part of the deal. Then followed a difficult time in our life together.

I had adapted to the catch-as-catch-can life of a freelancer, becoming a snapper-up of unconsidered trifles. I felt ill at ease in the role of consultant, usually telling clients how they could solve their problems without my help. I developed a public information strategy for a section of Environment Canada, taught two courses in community development at the Nova Scotia College of Art and Design, served as executive director of the Nova Scotia Association of Optometrists from 1978 to 1987, founded *The Atlantic Provinces Book Review* (now *Atlantic Books Today*), wrote five books on

Canadian history for an American publisher, produced a cable programme on offshore oil and gas development for the National Film Board, served as managing editor of *Axiom*, a short-lived regional magazine, published three "northerns" (murder mysteries set in Canada's north) and a thriller on the Halifax Explosion of 1917 and did a lot of freelance writing for a range of publications.

I continued my research on community development in Canada, Britain and elsewhere. In 1986, I spent a month in Wales at the invitation of the Wales Council for Voluntary Action, visiting community ventures and giving seminars. I taught public participation at the Banff School of Management and helped to set up the MBA in Community Economic Development at the University College of Cape Breton (now Cape Breton University). I taught summer courses there and served as a researcher/writer for *The Third Option*, a CD-ROM on community-based development produced by the college.

I learned to avoid investing my identity in my assignments. Journalists saw me as an academic while academics thought I was a journalist. My main interest, like Pat's, was to keep on learning.

When she lost her job with *The Southender* and *The Westender*, which she had run with very few resources, Pat lost part of her identity. She applied, without success, for other jobs. In her diary she recorded sending her resume to a company seeking an editor for newspaper flyers, lamenting that she had been the editor of a glossy magazine, then of papers printed on newsprint and now was hoping to edit flyers. In time, Pat adapted to her new status, doing freelance editing for organizations, serving as secretary of the Arts Advisory Council and becoming a member of the senate of the Atlantic School of Theology. Neither of us was very good at selling our services.

We enjoyed living in Halifax, a walkable city, and had a wide circle of friends. I worked out at a gym each morning while Pat walked around Point Pleasant Park with a friend, relishing the sights and sounds of this tamed wilderness. We took part in voluntary organizations, Pat with the Heritage Trust of Nova Scotia, editing a book of stories by people who had renovated heritage homes. *Affairs with Old Houses* appeared in 1999. I served on the board of the Sea Venturers' Society, a sail-training venture. Pat organized the book tables at the annual yard sales of St. George's Anglican Church, although she was not a member of the congregation.

In 1989, I received a grant from the Social Sciences and Research Humanities Council, as a private scholar, to continue my research on community development. Three years later, I was awarded the first Canada Council "A" grant for non-fiction to work on my book *The Lichen Factor*, about symbiosis in development.

And Pat became a property owner and an exemplary landlady.

In 1985, after the birth of Peter, our only grandson, Fiona broke up with her husband then divorced him. In 1993, she married Carl Smith whose chronic heart condition prevented him from doing steady work. To ensure that our daughter and her family had a roof over their heads, Pat bought a four-unit apartment building near Thorndean. She treated her tenants well, even allowing two impoverished students to leave without paying their last two months' rent.

Two of the tenants, Trevor and Linda, worked as chefs. One evening in January 1994, two plainclothes police officers came to our door. They informed us that Trevor was growing pot and offered Pat two options. She could give them the keys to the apartment and Trevor's unit — or they would break down the doors. Pat handed over the keys. The cops busted Trevor, who spent six months in jail. After his release, Pat asked him how he enjoyed his time inside. "It was wonderful!" he replied. "They put me in the kitchen and I livened up the food. The other inmates were sorry to see me leave."

Pat later sold the apartment building and bought a condominium unit for Fiona and her family. She handled all the transactions herself — something I never could have done and for which I admired Pat immensely.

In 1990, we worked together on *Nova Scotia*, a volume in Grolier's "Discover Canada" series, a supplementary school text. We made real money on this one and split the royalties. After joining Canadian Executive Services Organization (CESO) and undertaking assignments in Slovakia, Nain and with First Nations communities, I suggested to the president that I write a book on it — as a volunteer. Pat, as editor, was paid for her services. We had an interesting time meeting volunteers in Nova Scotia, Ottawa, Montreal and Toronto and collecting their stories. The resulting book, *Sharing a Lifetime of Experience: The CESO Story*, appeared in 1997.

I never learned how helpful Pat had been to others. Recommended for a position as editor of the *Dal News* at Dalhousie University, she passed on the offer to Roma Arsenault who wrote, "Many years later Pat went to bat for me again. Formac Publishing asked Pat to edit *The Haligonians* [profiles of prominent, deceased residents] but she didn't really want the job. Again I got the job thanks to Pat. I really loved working on that book, and it was only because of Pat that I got to do it. She was a great help...

regularly [walking] to our place…to make suggestions for subjects to write about and for writers."

The Haligonians was published in 2005. By that time, Pat had found a focus for her research and writing in recovering the story of James Forman, the first owner of Thorndean. As cashier, a position equivalent to vice-president, he tallied up the day's takings at the Bank of Nova Scotia and put the cash in the safe. Sometime after 1838, when he moved into Thorndean, and 1870, he skimmed off over $300,000 of the bank's money — about $3 or 4 million today. Forman fancied himself an entrepreneur. He invested in a builder who consistently lost money by underbidding on contracts. Forman tried, without success, to smuggle goods into the southern states during the American Civil War.

In 1992, Pat spent six weeks in Britain, doing research and visiting some of Forman's descendants. Pat worried how they would react on learning about the "bent banker," as one of them called him. They were delighted to have a roguish ancestor and treated Pat royally on her visits to them; several of them even came to Halifax. We entertained them in the house in which their ancestors had lived.

From 1992 onwards, Pat, after her early-morning walks in Point Pleasant Park, would vanish into the Public Archives of Nova Scotia to dig into the history of Halifax in the nineteenth century. James Forman became like a member of our family. One day, Pat returned from the archives, her eyes aglow: "He played the cello!"

Although the bent banker was fired, he was not prosecuted.

With his wife, Margaret Ann, he went to Londonderry, a mining town in Nova Scotia, to live with their son, Robert. The couple moved to London in 1872, where James died two years later.

We visited St. Anne's Square, their last address, in the centre of which stood the ugliest church in London, surrounded by hedges bedecked with barbed wire. Margaret Ann returned to Halifax to live with her son, Robert, dying in 1878. Later generations of Formans became railway engineers and admirals in the British navy.

James Forman must have been very attached to Thorndean, as his ghost has been seen here. Pat's book, *Banker, Builder, Blockade Runner*, published by Gaspereau Press in 2002, a meticulous piece of research and writing, places Forman in the context of his times, presenting a vivid picture of business and family life in Halifax in the middle of the nineteenth century.

Brian Forman, the great great grandson of James, wrote, "All Pat's work on the Formans of Halifax developed new bonds which would never have happened but for her. Her book was well read by over 35 Formans and other descendants of the King-Halls."

Travels

We both travelled a lot, on our own and together. Away from home, Pat became much more relaxed and uninhibited. I never discovered the reason for this, one of the mysteries about this woman I loved so deeply and dearly.

We visited Combermere, an intentional religious community in Ontario, and The Community of Christ the Sower, a similar venture in England. We went twice to Hay-on-Wye in Wales and browsed in its thirty-five bookstores.

We seldom did touristy things on our travels, being content to walk, hand-in-hand, around Venice, Rome,

Chester and elsewhere. We took the Helen Forrester Walk in Liverpool, named for the Canadian writer who told how her family fell from the middle class into poverty in the 1930s.

In Rome, Pat and I followed the story of *Tosca* from the Church of Sant' Andrea Della Valle to the palace of Baron Scarpia and across the Tiber to the Castel San Angelo, once the tomb of the emperor Hadrian. We walked up the ramp to the terrace from which Tosca throws herself at the end of the opera and laughed as we recalled a performance where the heroine, landing on a trampoline, bounced up again. We ate in a restaurant in the vaults of Pompey's theatre, the site of the murder of Julius Caesar, had a picnic at the Villa Giulia, which houses the Etruscan Museum and wandered around the Forum.

We had a stroke of luck one summer. After tramping and busing around the West Country of England in a wet summer, Pat decided to visit her sister in Rome. A travel agent told us that, for what it would cost Pat to fly there, we could have a week in a hotel. We discovered on reaching Rome that the staff there were on strike and moved to the Giulia Cesare, a "Belle-Epoque Palace," according to a guidebook.

Early each morning, we slipped out of the hotel and headed for the Janiculum Hill. We paid homage here to Anita Garibaldi, wife of the liberator of Italy. A statue shows her astride a horse, a pistol in one hand, a baby under her arm. From a nearby parapet we watched and listened as the sun touched the ochre walls of the Eternal City. We found a bench at the top of the Capitoline Hill, near where Edward Gibbon thought up his idea of a book on the decline and fall of the Roman Empire. We sat here, silent and content in each other's company, for a long time overlooking the

Forum. As the day warmed and the heat became heavy, we walked back to the hotel and made love in the afternoon.

We came to know Rome well. While walking along the Ponte Cestio from the Isola Tiberina, a car almost grazed Pat. She turned, gave the driver the finger, and shouted, "*Stupido!*" I was very proud of her.

On a wet, tree-dripping day, we visited Farrington Gurney, the village in the middle of nowhere to which Pat and her family had been evacuated after the blitz on Bath. There was "no there there" in this undistinguished rural community. We tramped along damp lanes until a welcome bus took us back to Bath.

We made another pilgrimage in 1997, to Carcassonne, in search of the family with whom Pat had stayed as an *au pair*. Many times she had told me of cassoulet, the delicious regional specialty. We ordered it on our first night in the hotel, but could not finish the enormous dish placed before us.

Pat and I wandered around the old medieval city of Carcassonne. Returning from it one evening, we looked back and saw the walls and towers bathed in floodlights, turning old Carcassonne into a shining city on a hill.

Memories of our travels together helped me to make connections with Pat during her dementia, as she retained some long-term memory. When I recalled the "*Stupido!*" incident, Pat would smile. When I spoke about wandering over Arthur's Seat in Edinburgh and of a wonderful stay in the Old Waverly in that city, I seemed to touch a chord of memory in Pat.

Two of Pat's journeys proved difficult for her. In 1987, she experienced "the most terrible thing that had ever happened to me." I believe Pat, as the elder sister, had to care for her siblings because of her mother's involvement with St. John's Ambulance, and so saw herself as responsible for their welfare. Annette, her youngest sister with whom we stayed in Rome, left her Italian husband and took up with an American professor. In the summer of 1987, she travelled to Maine to sort out their relationship. On the day after her arrival, Annette, who was not wearing a seatbelt, was fatally injured in a car accident. Pat went to be with her as she died in a hospital in Maine.

In 1998, Pat flew to Victoria to care for our daughter Annette — named for her aunt — after she came out of hospital. Serving in the Canadian Forces with a helicopter squadron in Esquimault, Annette had been misdiagnosed with irritable bowel syndrome. Unhappy love affairs and some difficult postings had hardened Annette. She treated Pat shabbily, demanding that she pay for her own food. When Annette's problem was identified as colorectal cancer, we flew out to be with her in February 2001.

Severe illnesses seem to affect people in two ways. A friend whose husband developed multiple sclerosis told me that, confined to a wheelchair, he became a tyrant in their last three years together. Annette became the kind, gentle person we had known when she was growing up. Her sister Fiona spent a week with her and told us, "Annette has become the sister I always wanted." On our visit, we had a wonderful time with Annette and spoke to her doctors. They tried to offer us hope, but it became obvious that — as with dementia — nothing could be done for Annette.

Her cancer went on its remorseless way.

When next we visited her, in August 2001, she was confined to bed in her apartment. In October, Annette entered the Victoria Hospice, a wonderful, peaceful place, where she would end her days. Our daughter endeared herself to all she met with her positive and cheerful attitude, politeness and the comfort she gave to others.

While a friend and I sat with her on an evening in March 2002, Annette said, "I can't take any more of this," repeating the words again and again. Pat and I spent the night of March 23 sleeping in her room, then she and a friend went in search of breakfast. I stayed with Annette, who was sleeping. Quite suddenly, she woke up, said, "Hi, Dad!" and died without a trace of fear. Annette left this life as she had lived, on her own terms, as the slight smile on her face told us.

When Pat returned to Annette's room, she was devastated at not being present at the moment of our daughter's death. Whenever Annette phoned with bad news, she always told me it first "so as not to upset Mum." We rationalized that our daughter died as she did to spare Pat's feelings. But, as I was to learn when Pat died, no matter how you rationalize the death of a loved one as "being for the best," you cannot escape the emotional toll it takes on you. And Pat found it hard to forgive herself for not being with Annette when she died.

In the fall of 2003, I went to Lesotho in southern Africa as a volunteer to examine the possibilities of establishing a master's degree in community economic development at the National University. A few days earlier, Hurricane Juan roared through Halifax, flooding streets, downing trees, knocking out power. Pat had problems with her short-term memory at this point, but I had no qualms about leaving her alone in a darkened house.

She would never have thought about asking me to cancel my trip, knowing how important were my commitments to the people who arranged it. Pat survived ten days without power, with help from our daughter and her friends. I never heard her complain about her ordeal.

By this time, our passion for each other had been complemented by a sense of loving companionship. We lived out what Antoine de Saint-Exupery, one of Pat's favourite authors, had learned: "Life has taught us that love does not consist of gazing at each other but in looking together in the same direction."

We had a very comfortable home, enough money to meet our needs, many friends and lots of interesting things to do.

Then Pat developed dementia and our lives changed.

The disease came like a thief in the night, without warning, afflicting the woman I loved, who had earned four university degrees and kept her mind busy throughout our married life.

As Pat's dementia worsened, I discovered one true thing: My love for her, and hers for me, would carry us through, form the foundation of our changed relationship and help us to cope with the strange, confusing world into which we plunged.

Chapter Five
Our Lifelong Love Affair

The point of a marriage is not to create a quick commonality by tearing down all boundaries; on the contrary, a good marriage is one in which each partner appoints the other to be the guardian of his solitude, and thus they show each other the greatest possible trust.

Rainer Maria Rilke

The romantic view of marriage portrays two people falling in love, taking vows and living happily ever after. The reality today is quite different, couples living together for a while then breaking up, half the marriages in North America ending in divorce. Anthropologists call this sort of thing "serial polygamy."

Is it possible for two people to love each other with equal

passion, to sustain that relationship throughout their lives, to become one while retaining their individuality?

A verse I picked up, source unknown, tells how I felt about Pat: "If equal affection cannot be, Then let the more loving one be me."

When we married, I told Pat, "You'll be angry, frustrated and often displeased with me. But you'll never be bored."

We lived in Montreal in the early winter of 1960. Soon after learning of Paul Walker's death in California, I became blind drunk at a party. A friend levered me into his bed. Waking up around two in the morning, stone cold sober, I looked around for my new wife. I could find no sign of her. Pat had left me to the good care of a friend with whom I had shared a tent in the Arctic. Seething with rage, I walked back to the apartment and banged on the door. Pat had decided to forgive me and be the understanding wife when I showed up. She opened the apartment door. I snarled, "What the hell do you mean, abandoning me?" Brushing past her, I collapsed into bed and sulked for a day.

An appropriate start for a wonderful, passionate relationship!

Strangers when we married, we learned over the years to deal with each other's shortcomings, quirks and peculiarities. Each of us had great drive, a lust for life, a fierceness to develop our individual potential, to keep on learning.

Separateness and Oneness

For one human being to love another human being: that is perhaps the most difficult task that

*has been entrusted to us, the ultimate test, the final
test and proof, the work for which all other work is
merely preparatory.*

Rainer Maria Rilke

Struggling for oneness, we recognized that we were different people. Even as our love for each other became deeper
and more satisfying, we remained a mystery to each other.
In February 2002, when Pat was in Victoria, I wrote to her,
"At times you seem to be a mystery to me — as I'm sure I
am to you. There is in you a sense of unfulfilled potential,
something beyond the here and now. I was surprised to hear
you say, some weeks ago, that you had little confidence in
yourself... We are an odd couple, my love, both very indi-
vidualistic yet with a strong sense of 'we.'"

Friends saw us as Pat and Jim or Jim and Pat, insepar-
able, never apart, close as the proverbial peas in the pod. Yet
at times, Pat appeared to me as if she stood behind a glass
wall and it took me time to accept this image, to see her as
a separate person from me. Our lives converged at times,
diverged at others. While at *Atlantic Insight*, Pat told me
that relatives of staff could not write for it. I knew this to be
untrue and resented it until I recognized the claim as part of
Pat's desire to have a separate identity and role in life.

In time we became attuned to each other's moods,
learned to respect them, doing together what we enjoyed
doing together, the most obvious being making love, which
was always pleasant and sometimes quite spectacular. Before
Pat developed dementia, we had become so close, especially
when we travelled together, that I hardly had a sense of Pat
as a separate being. Yet this closeness did not prevent us

from following our individual and particular pursuits. Pat did not ask for my help while writing her book on James Forman and I did not offer it.

Pat and I had solitary natures. Paradoxically, this brought us close. Friendly to all we met, we were not particularly sociable, finding in each other all we needed for our happiness. This self-reliance helped and hindered in caring for Pat in her last years.

I never discovered the source of Pat's penchant for solitude, but it may have had something to do with her romantic nature. Romanticism tends to encourage its followers to see themselves as solitary figures in a landscape, alone and palely loitering. In Pat's copy of Wordsworth's poems, she underlined his words written on the banks of the river Wye above Tintern Abbey as he observed "these beauteous forms:" "That on a wild secluded scene impress/Thoughts of more deep seclusion."

My solitary nature arose, in part, from the year I spent in Oldmeldrum after being evacuated there in 1939. I had nothing in common with the other school kids. They mocked my name — "Shallots!" — and ostracized me. My outsider status made me a scapegoat for the follies of my fellow students. If the teacher left the class, it descended into chaos. Mr. Mudie, the principal, dashed in to establish order. The only voice he could hear above the babble was mine, with its marked "scouse" accent. So I was hauled out and strapped. By the end of the school year, when I returned to Liverpool, I had a Scottish accent so thick that my father could not understand what I was saying.

My maiden aunts, whom I addressed by their first names, created a safe, secure home for me. I went on long walks by myself, equipped with a "piece" (sandwich) and instructions to be back in time for tea; the aunts never worried about their ten-year-old charge. I roamed the countryside, climbed Bennachie, the mountain that dominates the skyline, and wandered along country lanes empty of cars.

My solitary nature turned me into a reader. I took forty books with me on each of my Arctic ventures to keep my mind active in the white stillness of Northern Ellesmere Island. In the summer of 1958, I spent ten days alone on the Gilman Glacier with only a dog team for company and never felt lonely.

In the early days of our marriage, I tried to determine why Pat did what she did, thought as she did. She reacted angrily to my questions, accusing me of "psychoanalyzing" her. So I stopped doing this. When you love someone, acceptance is better than understanding.

As Shakespeare put it in Sonnet 116,

> *Let me not to the marriage of true minds*
> *Admit impediments, love is not love*
> *Which alters when it alteration finds,*
> *Or bends with the remover to remove.*
> *O no, it is an ever-fixed mark*
> *That looks on tempests and is never shaken.*

And we had plenty of tempests in our relationship!

I admired Pat as a person for her many fine qualities and abilities. She had excellent taste, a flair for clothes, colour and design that I lacked, and always looked well groomed, smart and elegant. In contrast, I usually look like an unmade bed and wore clashing colours that horrified Pat. She had a glad grace — not one of my attributes — and a charm of which she was seemingly unaware. A dental technician about to retire loaded Pat up with floss and other goodies. An apartment manager found Pat a three-bedroom apartment in a full building. Finding us stranded on the outskirts of Glasgow, a taxi driver took us into the centre of the city and refused payment. The staff of the medical facilities who cared for Pat, with one or two exceptions, delighted in dealing with her. She never complained and always thanked them for what they did for her. Doctors' records refer to "this very pleasant lady."

Through tensions and turmoil, crises and contentment, arguments and reconciliations, days of delight and moments of despair, Pat and I had a wonderful sense of Oneness at times, becoming the completion of each other. We bought a replica of the Lewis chess set, playing until we became bored from knowing each other's moves too well. Pat made an excellent black forest cake (*schwarzwaldtorte*). Walking through a liquor store, we spotted a wine labeled "Black Forest Girl." We both spluttered "Schwarzwaldtart" and dissolved in laughter. Without knowing it, we each kissed our dead daughter farewell with the same words: "Good night, sweet princess. And flights of angels sing thee to thy rest!"

Pat had known what life at the bottom of society, as a servant, was like. She had abundant agape, loving kindness, towards outsiders. On our Saturday morning walks down Spring Garden Road, Pat would stop and chat with Jean, a beggar woman, who told us of her many afflictions. Pat would listen intently, radiating concern, and I could see this troubled woman felt better for this. She refused to take money from us, but I always insisted she do so. Louise, a large, untidy street lady, smiled when she saw Pat, who always greeted her warmly and gave her something. When I told her of Pat's death she made a clumsy attempt to embrace me.

Pat never met a cat or a dog in the time of her early dementia without greeting and chatting with it. I said, "You've always been fond of dumb animals." She smiled and replied, "I married you, didn't I?"

I injected playfulness into our relationship. On our summer walks, I'd point out a flower: "Your favourite — impatiens." I put up a poster showing two kittens: "Be patient. God isn't finished with me yet." And to the tune of the Beatles' song "Yesterday," I'd sing, "Pussycats make such lovely gloves and furry hats." If I knew that Pat would be phoning me, I'd answer *Pronto* (Italian) or *Zur Befehl* (German). She'd laugh and say, "One day it won't be me." This happened, leaving one bewildered caller wondering if he had the right number.

We both worked with words, and this can be enormously frustrating. As T. S. Eliot put it, "Words strain, crack, and sometimes break… Decay with imprecision, will not stay in place,/Will not stay still." We talked a lot about words and language as we struggled to put black on white, each in our own way. Writers, journalists and others of that ilk are given to trying to escape from the stress of creativity by drinking excessively, engaging in adultery, practicing infidelity and messing up their lives in other ways. We lived quiet lives.

Pat wrote in her diary on April 19, 1990, "I have decided that Jim and I are seen as rather boring people. Jim, especially, when we meet people casually on the street tends to keep his conversation at a fairly earnest level. I know I have very little facility for lighthearted conversation."

Martin Rumscheidt, Pat's thesis advisor at the Atlantic School of Theology, with whom I took courses, remembered "both Pat and you well as you were among the most interesting students I ever had. It was good to be in your company."

Pat and I never saw ourselves as "intellectuals" or as being "artsy." We loved classical music, theatre, good books and art and thought there was something comical about those who effused over them. This reaction stemmed from our British working-class upbringing and our dislike of pretension.

One heritage of our past bound us together and proved vital in dealing with Pat's dementia. We had been "properly brought up," never took each other for granted and made plentiful use of "thank you," "please" and "sorry" in our conversation. Dementia made Pat verbally abusive to me. When I blew my cool, I was rude to her. Most of the time we remained polite to each other and that eased relationships.

Pat had an innocence about her, a naiveté, a refreshing trust in others. She lacked the hard edges that marked my character, which she had done so much to smooth.

Roma Arsenault wrote about an incident when she worked with Pat at *Atlantic Insight*: "Upstairs, the guys in the art department...were growing marijuana in planters in front of the house. Pat took on the job of watering the plants, not knowing she was nurturing an illegal substance. We chuckled about it but kept mum."

Poetry

Poetry is the spontaneous overflow of powerful feelings: it takes its origin from emotion recollected in tranquility.

William Wordsworth

Pat and I loved poetry, having imbibed large quantities of it in high school. Pat studied the Victorians and Romantics at Sir George Williams University, telling me how she and others spilled out of the classes, talking excitedly about what they had just learned. She had a well-worn copy of Earl Wavell's *Other Men's Flowers,* an unusual bouquet put together by a soldier. I favoured the Moderns, Eliot, Auden, MacNeice; the war poets, Owen, Sassoon; Shakespeare's sonnets, Housman, Omar Khayyam and the like. Poetry formed a bond between us, giving me insights into Pat's nature that I could never discover in any other way.

During our courtship, Pat invited me to stay for a weekend at the farm her sister Marie managed near Varennes, on the south shore of the St. Lawrence. I have a vivid recollection of Pat standing at a picture window, gazing into the darkness, reciting the last lines of Matthew Arnold's "Dover Beach:"

> *Ah, love, let us be true*
> *To one another!*
> *For the world which seems*
> *To lie before us like a land of dreams,*
> *So various, so beautiful, so new,*
> *Hath really neither joy, nor love, nor light,*
> *Nor certitude, nor peace, nor help for pain:*
> *And we are here as on a darkling plain*
> *Swept with confused alarms of struggle and flight*
> *Where ignorant armies clash by night.*

This poem echoed a streak of sorrow, of pessimism, in Pat.

As a romantic, she had continually to contend with realities that did not match her imaginings. I was more of an optimist than Pat. Before leaving for the High Arctic in 1957, I took part in a study to determine the kind of people best suited to work there. Shown a photo of a man at an open high window, I was asked, "What does this picture say to you?" I replied, "He's looking out at a new day, full of optimism about what it will bring." A pessimist, presumably, would have said the bloke was about to chuck himself out of the window.

Pat had a mystical chord in her nature, which emerged from her love of Walter de la Mare's poem "The Listeners," which she knew by heart. A man on horseback gallops up to an isolated house in a forest clearing: "'Is there anybody there?' said the Traveller,/Knocking on the moonlit door."

No one replies for "only a host of phantom listeners" hears "that voice from the world of men." The traveller shouts, "'Tell them that I came and no one answered/That I kept my word.'" The listeners hear the horseman depart: "And how the silence surged softly backwards,/When the plunging hoofs were gone." Why did this poem fascinate Pat?

She wrote in a notebook, "'The Listeners,' one of my favourite poems I can recite from beginning to end. It has always had a powerful emotional hold on me — if offers infinite possibilities for wonder at its meaning, origin."

She added another, unattributed line from a poem: "Look thy last on all things lovely every hour." And followed it with

Eyes bid ears
Hark;
Ears bid eyes
Mark...
Heart bids mind
Wonder:

Mind bids heart
Ponder.

(From *"Two Deep Clear Eyes"*)

I would recite to Pat the opening lines from Shakespeare's Sonnet 18 to tell her how I felt about her: "Shall I compare thee to a summer's day? Thou art more lovely and more temperate."

When she worried about aging, I would again resort to the immortal bard: "To me fair friend you can never be old."

Pat would respond by quoting the next line, surely one of the worst any poet ever wrote — "For as you were when first your eye I eyed" — and we would laugh.

As a freelancer, forever looking for a way to earn an honest dollar, I would oft bewail "my outcast state." Then I would think of my life with Pat and the ending of Sonnet 29: "For thy sweet love remember'd such wealth brings,/That then I scorn to change my state with kings."

Pat's taste in art, which I shared, helped me to understand her — and myself. *Nighthawks*, Edward Hopper's painting of lonely people in an all-night diner, and his images of isolated people and houses, struck a responsive chord in Pat, as did the empty piazzas of de Chirico. On a visit to the National Gallery in London, Pat selected a print of Renoir's *The Umbrellas* to hang in our bedroom. A beautiful, sad-faced young woman, carrying a basket, stands on the left-hand side of the work. Behind her a crowd, all of whose members carry umbrellas, emphasizes the lost and lonely look of the woman who lacks one.

Poetry, our shared love of language, music and art forged links between us. Other aspects of our life kept us apart, gave us time and space we needed to follow our different interests and develop ourselves as individuals.

Anxiety

The fear of life is the favourite disease of the twentieth century.

William Lyon Phelps

Pat had two characteristics with which she struggled throughout her life and with which I found difficult to deal: she was a procrastinator and a worrier. I am neither. Every summer, as the sun poured through the window of our south-facing kitchen, Pat would say, "We should get blinds." Since the house was her domain, I readily agreed. The summer sun still floods our blindless kitchen. Pat's book *Banker, Builder, Blockade Runner* acknowledges my help "for nagging me into finishing it."

Pat's worrying worried me because I could do so little to assuage it. I told her, often, that if they ever made worrying an Olympic sport, she'd win a gold for Canada.

Where these feelings of anxiety originated I never did determine. Losing her job at *The Southender* at the age of fifty-nine had a marked impact on her, for she enjoyed running the community newspapers. Under the serene and tranquil front Pat presented to life lay a great deal of inner turmoil. She developed a marvelous capacity for picking herself up after mental and physical distress. "Elegant, with a core of steel," is how Fiona remembers her mother.

The words of Rilke echoed through our relationship: "A

merging of two people is an impossibility, and where it seems to exist, it is a hemming-in, a mutual consent that robs one party or both parties of their fullest freedom and development."

Pat and I never hemmed each other in, for, quite unconsciously, we saw ourselves as the guardians of each other's solitude. We recognized that, even though we loved each other, we each had battles to fight on our own.

On July 30, 1986, while reading Charles Williams's *All Hallows Eve*, which features a character with an urge to control others, Pat had a disturbing moment of truth: "I saw that I have always sought to dominate my environment — my parents, my friends, my children, and even Jim who, thank God, is not to be dominated… I realize that this must have made life very stressful for Annette and Fiona."

She blamed herself for Annette bullying Fiona (and Dino) and for Fiona's lack of confidence.

We did not discuss this revelation. Had we done so, I would have assured Pat that what she blamed herself for could be explained in other ways.

Themes of struggle, striving, seeking and worrying pervade Pat's diary entries, which tended to be irregular. She wondered whether her prayers were turning into reflections of "my psychological shortcomings." In June 1991, she expressed alarm that her memory was "declining alarmingly." On September 26 in that year, she became, as she put it, "pissed off" with me.

According to astrology, we Capricorns are perfectionists. And I was stupid in dealing with Pat's worries and concerns.

My male mentality led me to believe that if you have a problem, you do something about it; you do not brood over it. I too often blew my cool over Pat's behaviour, failing to understand why she did what she did. I would assure her that there was "nothing personal" in my criticisms. Pat needed comfort and support when she became upset — not sermons.

I forget the incident that pissed Pat off in 1991. She wrote in a diary, "He's an intelligent, bright individual but I could talk for an hour and still not be able to get through to him that his double standard of behaviour is ridiculous. Much as I love Thorndean, if I could afford to move out, I would. I love him, but can't take the idiotic pattern of behaviour much longer."

A week after that entry, Pat wrote, "Once again, all is well between Jim and Me — a little better if anything." A friend, married for sixty years, told me he never had an argument with his wife. Pat and I had a lot in common, but we reacted to the slings, arrows and flowers of bad and good fortune in different ways. The result was some monumental rows.

We always made up after a few days of moody silence, forgetting what had caused the breach between us, returning to laughter and good companionship.

Pat was more forgiving of my faults — real and imagined — than I was of hers. She complained once to a friend — the only time she did so — that I bought too many books. I believed it impossible to have too many books, and Pat was no slouch when it came to acquiring them; she would leave the St. George's book sales with armfuls of volumes. When we ran out of bookcases, Pat sent me out to buy some at a private sale. I came back with the bookcases — and the books that had been on them.

Pat was not pleased. But she was not surprised.

Some of Pat's anxieties may have stemmed from what appears to have been the precarious state of her family's finances while she was growing up. Working-class people fear falling into the pit of poverty. I also was acutely aware of how important it was to retain one's dignity by ensuring financial independence.

Aging added to Pat's anxieties.

Women internalize their emotions and are too prone to criticize what they see as their shortcomings. Pat paid meticulous attention to her complexion, dress and appearance. She would see something she liked in a quality-clothing store, wait until it went on sale, then snap it up. I told her often what a smart, good-looking broad she was.

And I found myself in a Catch-22 situation.

On August 13, 1992, Pat wrote about "...my image of myself, which is disintegrating. This is because of my increasing overbite...mixture of vanity and low self-esteem. It's absolutely impossible to communicate with Jim about my fears. He dismisses my concern about my appearance but he actually exacerbates it unconsciously by his compliments on my appearance, especially when we go to any social gathering. 'You were the best-looking woman there,' is typical of his comments. By this time next year there will be no way in which he can make such a statement."

On August 16, 1992, Pat recorded a "mind-numbing depression" and thought it was "God nudging me to be less concerned with outward appearances."

In 1992, Pat handed in her master of theology thesis and began research on the book on James Forman, recording that she was "filled with optimism." On January 29, 1993, she was moved by "one particularly endearing inscription" on a Greek tomb while watching John Rohmer's TV programme *Seven Wonders of the World*. The parents of a dead child ask Charon, who conveys the souls of the dead across the river

Styx, "to help our little boy out of the boat. He does not walk very well and his shoes are new." Pat's response to these words revealed how, despite anxiety and depression, she remained the dear, kind, caring person whom I loved so much but for whom I could do so little.

On March 31, 1995, Pat wrote in her diary about "depression — inability to make decisions, inability to stop feeling I should be controlling the world around me, inability to rid myself of turning problems into obsessions." On April 26, she prayed, "God, save me from myself."

Pat spoke to me of her acedia, the noonday devil, sloth, laziness, one of the seven deadly sins. A prayer I found among her papers showed how, with typical resilience, she dealt with her anxieties and fears: "O God, I am feeling anxious and afraid, I ask for your help to calm me down, to do my best with you beside me and within. With you I know all things are possible. So I am claiming this as your promise to me now. I'm going forward aware that I am not alone. I will fear no evil for you are with me indeed. Thank you. Amen."

In 1995, Pat officially retired when she received Old Age Security and Canada Pension Plan payments. Combined with income from the sale of her apartment building, they helped Pat to feel financially secure. In that year, we had a splendid holiday in British Columbia, visiting old friends and making new ones. The Forman book kept her busy until 2002.

In 2003, after Annette died, Pat had five sessions with a psychologist (at $120 an hour) to deal with her anxiety and depression. She had been prescribed clonazepam to help her cope with them, but weaned herself off the drug. On June 15, 2003, she wrote in her diary, "Felt ghastly in the evening — utterly overwhelming feeling of losing control. Jim helped me over it." This may have been a reaction to withdrawal from clonazepam. We never placed much reliance on pills and learned over the years that the side effects of some drugs were worse than the conditions they claimed to treat.

I did what I could to help Pat deal with her demons, without hemming her in or trying, in my clumsy way, to slay them. Before and after she developed dementia, I did all I could to cheer her up, play the fool, make her smile or laugh. I drew upon a rich store of jokes, poems and songs that I had accumulated, some of them rather rude.

As Pat lay abed in the morning, I would quote the opening stanza of *The Rubaiyat of Omar Khayyam*:

> *Awake! for Morning in the Bowl of Night*
> *Has flung the Stone that puts the Stars to Flight:*
> *And lo! the Hunter of the East has caught*
> *The Sultan's Turret in a Noose of Light.*

If we hit an unavoidable snag, I would recite lines from *Albert and the Lion*. After the lion eats Albert, the story goes:

> *"Let's look on the bright side," said Father,*
> *"Wot can't be 'elped must be endured;*
> *Each cloud 'as a silvery lining*
> *And we did 'ave young Albert insured."*

We would laugh, decide we would endure whatever happened to us and go on with our lives.

Pat told me, several times, of her dreams about sitting on the toilet. I suggested they meant that she was ridding herself of waste, superfluous matters cluttering up her life, dumping disturbing thoughts. This seemed to make sense to her.

Before she developed dementia, Pat had learned to deal with her anxieties and depression. A diary entry, after an attack of depression, noted, "This too will pass." Pat took communion regularly, started doing tai chi and much enjoyed it, threw the I Ching every month and recorded what it told her, read books on labyrinths as spiritual journeys and made notes on them, learned Italian, meditated, sketched, checked astrological forecasts, made beautiful quilts for our home and for friends, prayed for those in distress (intercessionary prayer) and did other things that gave her quiet comfort. Pat always felt that she should be doing more than she was doing, despite my suggestions that she take life a little easier as we aged. An entry into her diary summed up her discontent: "I do not have enough that absorbs my attention whether I will it or not."

Despite her oft-troubled thoughts and struggles with herself, Pat had a sense of profound spirituality about her on which others remarked.

Spirituality

> *Dust as we are, the immortal spirit grows*
> *Like harmony in music; there is a dark*
> *Inscrutable workmanship that reconciles*
> *Discordant elements.*

> *William Wordsworth*

It's difficult to articulate the essence of spirituality, a vague, nebulous term that describes ways of thinking and acting that play a large role in our lives. Spirituality shows us how to free ourselves from material concerns, opens us up to the wonders of the world, transcendence and humility, forces us to examine our relationships, inspires us to go beyond our smallness.

Pat had a problem common to those seeking to live a spiritual life in a materialistic world; she wondered if she was too attached to her dresses, the Staffordshire animals she collected and other worldly goods. Pat struggled to find a place in the formal structures of the Christian church for her spiritual quest. Finding none, she explored other ways of meeting them.

Pat never belonged to a congregation; such groups have been invaluable in supporting members dealing with dementia.

Feelings of restlessness, an inability to work or to pray, plagued Pat at times as she struggled between earthly and spiritual demands. Her curious religious upbringing may have had something to do with this. In Brighton and Bath she and her sisters had attended a convent school. On Sunday mornings, Pat went with her father to a high Anglican church. In the evenings a grandmother took her to a Foursquare Gospel meeting.

Throughout her life, Pat struggled with her belief and her unbelief. In the Gospel of Mark, the father of a boy possessed by a spirit tells Jesus, "I do have faith, but not enough. Help me to have more!" (9:24). In a diary entry on November 3, 1984, Pat wrote, "My openness to receiving God's grace is increasing." Pat slid back from time to time on her spiritual journey, picked herself up and continued the

quest for holiness, freedom from ambition and covetous-
ness, doing what she could for others.

My spiritual roots, unlike Pat's, did not lie in formal
religious structures. They arose from the camaraderie,
selflessness, courage and commitment that I experienced
and saw in wartime Britain. When the country stood alone
in 1940, Prime Minister Winston Churchill spoke of the
final triumph of good over evil when "the life of the world
[would] move forward into broad, sunlit uplands." We never
reached that place, but many people in Britain maintained
the sense of service that had brought us together in our time
of peril when the very existence of the nation hung in the
balance.

Growing up in Liverpool, I saw how religion divided
people. The family was loosely Church of England, and I
attended St. Simon and St. Jude on Sundays. Religion played
no part in our daily life. The Church of England of my youth
wallowed in guilt, fear, sin and the redemptive power of Jesus'
blood. The sermons bored me stiff. How could a man who
died two thousand years ago in a distant land take responsibility for my sins? Which were pretty minor and hardly worth
his attention, compared to the other evils in the world.

My Scottish aunts took me to the Church of Scotland up
the road in Oldmeldrum. This huge, pink barn had all the
charm of an aircraft hangar. Calvinism flourished here. This
harsh religion did little to stop people sinning, merely from
enjoying it.

On visits to the village in later years, I saw the church
turn into a huge chicken coop before disappearing and being
replaced by bungalows. The process struck me as a symbol
of the decline of organized religion. Rejecting it, I sought
sources of spirituality and religious inspiration elsewhere.

I have never been much interested in material things — except for books; much of my wardrobe comes from the Salvation Army.

A sixteenth-century poet, soldier, courtier and perfect gentleman and a modern novelist had a profound influence on my view of how I should live. Sir Philip Sidney, mortally wounded at Zutphen in the Low Countries in 1586, saw a suffering soldier lying nearby. He gave water offered to him to the man: "Thy necessity is greater than mine."

Somerset Maugham's *The Razor's Edge* also gave me ideas on living the good life. Larry Darnell, hero or anti-hero, serves as a pilot in World War I. A friend saves his life at the expense of his own, sending Larry on a quest to discover the roots of his being and to explore the mystery of the world. To our ears, it all sounds a bit New Age, but Maugham makes Larry believable and likeable. He comes from a good family, has a distinguished war record and is expected, after the war, to marry, settle down, take a job for life and become a member of the middle class. Larry refuses this destiny. He sets off in search of the Absolute, working in menial jobs, living simply, travelling to India, finding a guru, spending months in complete isolation. The book ends with Larry off somewhere, continuing his never-ending quest, finding happiness in a search for goodness in a depressing world. Maugham writes that Larry is without ambition, that he has a "glowing belief that ultimate satisfaction can only be found in the life of the spirit..." A rather good film of the novel, with Tyrone Power as Larry, came out in 1948, a rather bad one, with Bill Murray in the role, in 1984.

Finding nought for my comfort in Christianity, I read about Hinduism (too many gods), Islam, whose simplicity and austerity appealed to me, and Buddhism. I was attracted to Mahayana Buddhism, the "greater vessel," and the concept of the Bodhisattva who rejects nirvana to help others along their paths of salvation with wisdom and compassion. A life with few possessions attracted me, as did the Buddhist way of dealing with dualities and ambiguity. The western mind, schooled in rationalism and the division between mind and body, sees things in terms of either/or. People are either sane or crazy, of sound mind or not. The Buddhist concept of the self and the non-self is useful in dealing with ambiguous feeling while caring for a loved one. Pat, during her dementia, was there, with me, at times and absent at others. As her moods and behaviour changed, I "attached" myself to her when she needed me and "detached" myself from her when she took care of herself.

Someone claimed that Christianity brought the idea of sin and guilt into the world; sin originally meant "missing the mark," something we do all the time. A Jewish saying describes guilt as "the gift that keeps on giving."

Pat and I never discussed our religious beliefs. I never concerned myself with sin and guilt. If God is good — and He can't be otherwise — and loves His creation, then He gives us freedom to live and learn how to be fully human. If you truly love someone, you learn to suspend judgment about what they do, accept them as they are, respect their identity and integrity, make allowances for their weaknesses and shortcomings, while becoming aware of your own.

This theology may sound simple-minded, but it works for me, and proved important in caring for Pat. As a scientist, I developed a healthy skepticism about the world and those who inhabit it, taking nothing on trust, checking everything. Late in life, I came across the work of Gabriel Marcel, a French Christian existentialist philosopher who served as a stretcher-bearer in the First World War. He distinguished between problems and mysteries. A problem is "outside" you. It can be solved if you have the right physical and mental tools. You fill in a crossword by finding the right words. You assemble a jigsaw puzzle by putting the pieces in the right places to complete the whole. You don't solve mysteries. They are "inside" you. They don't have answers. You explore them throughout your life, striving to make sense of what is happening to you and to others. The causes of Alzheimer's and other dementias remain a mystery that is the subject of intensive research. Caring for a person with dementia, you have to learn to accept the mysteries of the strange ways in which he or she behaves.

Marcel made another seemingly simple observation: "The ticket collector is not the ticket collector." People have more dimensions to their beings than the labels we stick on them tell us. Pat was always a person in her own right, not just my wife, with dimensions of her character that I understood and others that baffled me.

My approach to spirituality moved outwards.

Pat's moved inwards.

She enjoyed being a member of the Anglican community at the Atlantic School of Theology, worshipping in the chapel, relishing the "psychic contagion" she experienced. AST, on whose senate she served after graduation, and whose newsletter she edited, proved to be a way station on Pat's spiritual journeying. Her master of theological studies thesis reflected this. It dealt with holistic ways of Christian life through which people live their faith in continual communion with God. *New Patterns of Christian Life* describes the origin and status of intentional religious communities, including Iona, Koinonia (from which sprang

Habitat for Humanity) and Sojourners. Pat drew attention to the resemblance they bear to Dietrich Bonhoeffer's concept of "religionless Christianity." The German Lutheran pastor, executed by the Nazis in April 1945, saw how the churches in his country accommodated themselves to Hitler and Nazism when the dictator took power in 1933. Bonhoeffer sought a life-affirming expression of Christianity, a form free of what he associated with religion.

As Pat put it, "I speculate that he could have come no closer to such an expression than one of the several types of Christian community profiled in this thesis: groups of Christians, united in their love of Christ and of humankind, their prayer and worship inextricably bound up with life in the world and their communion with each other."

Our two spiritual quests came together as I told Pat of my research and experience with people creating communities for personal and collective development. Between 1996 and 1999, our interests converged in a newsletter we issued. *Christian Community*, later *Community Connections*, linked spiritual and community development. We visited churches and cathedrals during our travels, enjoying evensong, singing the hymns of our childhood.

Pat started a spiritual journal on June 19, 1984, which I discovered after her death. She read and made notes on the works of Jim Wallis, Rollo May, Viktor Frankel (a favourite of mine), Monica Furlong, Judith Viorst (a strong influence), Madeleine L'Engel, Susan Howarth and other writers on spirituality and religion. Pat's notes, some on scraps of paper, continue to surface: "Courage is the capacity to meet the anxiety which arises as we achieve freedom" (Rollo May, *The Meaning of Anxiety*). From *Full Catastrophe Living* by Jon Kabat-Zinn, Pat copied out a list of what was needed to achieve it: "Non-judging, Patience, Beginner's Mind, Trust, Non-striving, Acceptance, Letting Go." Pat noted a poem by Judith Viorst, "The Pleasures of an Ordinary Life," that gave her comfort, for we never saw our lives, despite our spiritual strivings, as anything but ordinary. Pat relished the healing power of walking, quoting Thoreau: "An early morning walk is a blessing for the day." As she aged, Pat found more joy in her life as she learned to accept herself and our love grew stronger and deeper.

We became interested in the ideas of Carl Jung and explored them together and on our own. The concept of coming to terms with the dark side of our natures, our shadow, and integrating it into our lives appealed to us. This process, of acceptance of shortcomings and the demons that drive us, known as individuation, takes place later in life. We neither of us knew the source of our shadows, only that we each had one. As Jung put it, "To confront a person with his shadow is to show him his own light." Pat and I struggled, together and on our own, to confront our dark sides and to find our lights.

I had no name for Pat's luminous, spiritual quality until I came upon Yeats's poem, "When You Are Old," and recognized her "pilgrim soul." With this recognition came the realization that I, too, possessed one. And that Pat's loving presence in my life had done much to keep me going on my journey. Pilgrim souls, restless, forever questioning, need stars to guide them. And Pat was ever mine. I would often repeat to her when she questioned what she had done, "Nobody's perfect." She would reply with a quote from Browning: "Ah, but a man's reach must exceed his grasp/Or what's a heaven for?"

Pat's reach always exceeded her grasp, and I admired her for this, while wondering whether it contributed to her anxieties and the way she judged herself.

Looking back over our single and joint spiritual journeys, the words of T. S. Eliot come to mind:

We shall not cease from exploration
And the end of all our exploring
Will be to arrive where we started
And know the place for the first time.

Pat and I started our life together with love and a desire to learn about the world and ourselves. We did this with passion and enthusiasm in a life that sometimes frustrated us, but much more often refreshed, renewed and reinvigorated our love for each other.

Our last exploring took place during Pat's years with dementia. We remained content, most of the time, in each other's company. In her last months, Pat sat at the dining room table, a slight smile on her face, looking as serene and beautiful as ever. I knew she was no longer anxious and afraid, that her pilgrim soul was ending its journey and that she was at peace with herself and the world.

PART TWO
Foreground: The Long Goodbye

The progression of Alzheimer disease varies from person to person...

Day to Day, Alzheimer Society, August 2002

Caring for someone with dementia thrusts you into a world with aspects of the movie *Groundhog Day*. Time seems to stop as you are asked the same question, hour after hour, day after day. You recall the Monty Python dead parrot sketch as the sufferer denies what is obvious to you: "This is not my shoe!" Carers note the Alice in Wonderland feeling that comes over them as conversations take strange turns and things disappear down rabbit holes; I am still looking for a box of pens I bought six years ago. After difficult beginnings, you learn to adapt if you infuse all you do with love. But it is never easy.

Mary Geist quit her job as a radio news anchor and a promising career in the United States to help her mother care for her father after he developed Alzheimer's. She does not play down the frustrations, exhaustion and confusions of the role of caregiver. After helping her father to dress, she almost left the house wearing pyjamas. Geist's book, *Measure of the Heart*, resonates with the author's love for her father, who lived a full life. Like Pat, he was not difficult to care for. Geist quotes Henry Ward Beecher: "What the heart has once owned and had, it can never lose." A friend whose husband developed front temporal dementia assured me, "The heart knows better."

Heather Menzies, a Canadian writer, tells how difficult it can be if love is absent from a parental relationship. Memories of old injuries, insults and shortcomings surface during dementia. Menzies's mother, a dominating, controlling person, had made herself the centre of her home and of the lives of her children. Her daughter, in caring for her, had not only to cope with fear — "The prospect terrified me" — when her mother was diagnosed with Alzheimer's. She also had to deal with the emotional baggage from her past relationship with her. Menzies describes the erratic way in which her mother drove to see a doctor. And her stubborn response when told that she could no longer drive: "How can you know I am not a good driver?"

As well as being a carer, Menzies had an ill son and a leaky marriage. Somehow, as she tells in *Enter Mourning*, she found the strength and the wisdom to let go of the resentment she harboured against her mother. Menzies became a dutiful and caring daughter, aided by the contentment her mother felt in her last years.

In the years of her dementia, Pat remained the kind, loving person she had always been. From time to time, however, her anger surfaced and she called me nasty names. I never minded this. Where that anger originated I never discovered. One of the difficulties in dealing with people with dementia is the sudden emergence of behaviour that you have never experienced with them before that leaves you puzzled and dismayed. But whatever the behaviour, its roots lie in a past lost to the loved one and to you. The immediate reality is the only one, and you must learn how to cope with it.

Chapter Six
Discovering Dementia

When I left England in 1974, no one was talking about the disease.

Frena Gray-Davidson, *The Alzheimer's Sourcebook for Caregivers*

A newsletter from the Alzheimer Society tells of a man whose father suffered from a progressive, debilitating condition in the mid-1970s. He sent an article from *The Washington Post* on a "then little-known disease" to his mother. She showed it to the family doctor: Was this what her husband was suffering from? The physician chastised her for the self-diagnosis: "Alzheimer's disease is a very rare disease that affects people in their forties. Your husband is just getting old."

In truth, it is difficult to distinguish the loss of short-term memory, a normal part of aging, from early onset Alzheimer's.

You ask yourself, Why am I in this room? Where are my keys? What's that guy's name? Old people in the past were expected to go a bit barmy, to be "touched," to suffer from senile dementia as their brains "softened." *The Little Oxford Dictionary and Thesaurus* lists an astonishing number of synonyms for "mad:" insane, deranged, crazy, demented, lunatic, *non compos mentis*, unbalanced, unhinged, manic. Informal synonyms include out of your mind, nuts, round the bend, barmy, batty, bonkers. All cultures have words for those deemed to have lost their wits. In Scotland they are "dottled."

Yiddish speakers call sufferers *meshuggeneh*.

Madness has been a feature of human existence for an unknown number of years. Solon (c638–559 BCE), Greek lawgiver and philosopher, noted that impaired judgment in old age invalidated a will. As a disease of the aged, dementia reflects the lengthening lifespan, a sign of progress that has marked the last two hundred years. In 1800, average global life expectancy at birth was 28.5 years. In 2001, it stood at 66.6 years and is much higher in western nations.

In the past, those afflicted with dementia who became a danger to themselves and others were placed in institutions, locked up in back rooms and attics or cared for by their bewildered families.

Alzheimer's, named for the German physician who first identified it, was found in a patient in the late 1890s. Her worried husband brought her to see Dr. Alois Alzheimer (1864–1915) because of her strange behaviour. After her death, an autopsy revealed the characteristic plaques and tangles in the brain of what Alzheimer called pre-senile dementia. He published a full clinical and pathological description of the case in 1907.

In recent years, as people live longer, dementia has

become the basis of a growth industry in medicine and care-giving. Dementia results in more years lived with disability than stroke, heart disease and all forms of cancer. One in five Canadians over the age of forty-five provides care for seniors with long-term problems. Many of these older people not only suffer from Alzheimer's, but also what doctors refer to as comorbidity — other ailments. As the baby boomers, cradled in a culture of entitlement and instant gratification, age, the pressures to find a cure for Alzheimer's and other dementias will accelerate, as will the search for more effect-ive methods of caregiving and ensuring the best quality of life for sufferers. France and Japan are pioneers in this field, with emphasis on providing care in the home and in small facilities rather than in large institutions.

More than five hundred thousand Canadians over the age of sixty-five suffer from some form of dementia. If present trends persist, the number will rise to 1.1 million in 2038, and the cost of care increase to $153 billion a year from the present $8 billion. Like much of the data on dementia, these figures are informed guesses concealing the anguish, frustra-tion and damaged lives of sufferers and those who care for them. Dementia has been described as a global pandemic. An estimated thirty-five million people suffer from it, more than those afflicted with HIV/AIDS. By 2050, one person in eighty-five will have the mind-killing disease, making mock-ery of Browning's exultant "Grow old along with me! The best is yet to be." A quarter of those looking after people with dementia in Canada are seniors, living out their last days caring for loved ones.

Alzheimer's also afflicts those in their forties and fifties.

After sixty-five, the risk of dementia doubles every five years. Half of those who live to be over eighty-five will develop some form of dementia. Women appear particularly prone to Alzheimer's, making up 70 per cent of those afflicted by it.

The term *dementia* covers five main types of the disease, with Alzheimer's making up about 60–65 per cent of sufferers from it. The next most common category, depending on what you read, is either Lewys's body disease (sufferers also have Parkinson's) or vascular dementia caused by decreased cranial blood flow. They make up 20 per cent of dementias. Frontal/temporal dementia (Pick's disease, which renders those with it mute) and other forms caused by strokes comprise the balance.

Although CT scans of Pat's brain showed none of the characteristic patterns of Alzheimer's, she was diagnosed with it in 2009. She may have had vascular dementia or a combination of this and Alzheimer's. One of the many stumbling blocks in dealing with dementia is the impossibility of determining exactly what kind a sufferer has, except by an autopsy.

Mystery enshrouds dementia. No one knows what causes it.

Genetic factors almost certainly play a role in the development of dementia. The brains of those who die with Alzheimer's show clumps formed by excessive quantities of beta-amyloid, a protein. As the tangles spread, they block the functions of healthy neurons. Losing their ability to communicate through synapses, the minute gaps across which nerve impulses pass from one to the other, the neurons die. It is as if the links in a cellphone or a Blackberry become disconnected and the information they carry becomes distorted and unreadable. The brains of older people can atrophy with age, as Pat's did. Why these things happen in the most complex organ of the body continues to puzzle scientists.

The sole consolation for sufferers and carers is that dementia is a painless disease.

Drugs can slow down dementia, but no cure for it has been found nor is there any sign of one at this time.

The media now regularly feature news about dementia, which has become a stock part of movies, TV series and dramas. Shots show a sad-faced older person with a blank expression and unfocused eyes, images that contribute to the sense of hopelessness about the disease. In fact, many dementia sufferers can be lively and quite normal at times, as I discovered in caring for Pat.

Alzheimer's has its own month (January) and day (September 21) and an international organization that brings together seventy groups concerned with the disease, so that it has become shorthand for all kinds of dementia. DASNI (Dementia Advocacy and Support Network International) gives a voice to sufferers and those who care for them. The Canadian Alzheimer Society, founded in 1978, was the first national organization of its kind in the world. Canada also has a Dementia Action Network (CDAN).

There is an abundance of material on dementia and caregiving. The Canadian Alzheimer Society issues short, helpful brochures on these topics. Because every sufferer from dementia, and every caregiver, is an individual, it is difficult to generalize about the most effective way to cope with its onset and progress. Only too often, as I did, you learn something useful when it is too late to make use of it. Dealing with dementia involves endless learning and unlearning. The caregivers we hired from the Canadian Red Cross proved to be some of my best teachers.

Defining Dementia

Patients with dementia are not without feeling, understanding and humanity.

Kenneth Rockwood and Chris MacKnight,
Understanding Dementia

People with dementia do not cease to be human beings simply because something has gone wrong in their brains. They still have capacities for living full lives, for savouring small joys, for smelling the flowers.

The American Psychiatry Society describes the "essential feature of dementia" as "...[the] insidious onset and gradual progressive course for which all other specific causes have been excluded by the history, physical examination, and laboratory tests. The Dementia involves a multifaceted loss of intellectual abilities such as memory, judgment, abstract thought, and other higher cortical functions, and changes in personality and behavior."

The Bantam Medical Dictionary defines dementia as "A chronic and persistent disorder of behavior and higher intellectual function due to organic brain disease. It is marked by memory disorders, changes in personality, deterioration in personal care, impaired reasoning ability and disorientation."

The Oxford Companion to the Mind (1987) devotes three columns to dementia, quoting a book published in 1978 for its definition: "an acquired global impairment of intellect, memory and personality, without impairment of consciousness." It adds, "It follows that even severe dementia may not necessarily cause its sufferers any personal pain, depending on where and how he is cared for. If his environment is simple, cheerful and constant (i.e., unchanging) he may to all outward appearances (and on his own admission) be perfectly cheerful and contented."

This statement does something to alleviate the fear and distress that afflict family members when one of them is diagnosed with dementia. It also shifts the emphasis from attempts to cure it to efforts at creating the best possible quality of life for sufferers. This can be hard work, depending on the past relationships between them and those caring for them. Books and films like Nicholas Sparks' *The Notebook* and *Away from Her*, based on an Alice Munro story, present a sanitized view of dementia; they ignore the awful aspects of the disease.

Still Alice, a bestseller by Lisa Genova, a neuroscientist, contains a great deal of useful information on Alzheimer's. It tells the story of Alice Howland, a Harvard cognitive psychology professor, an expert in linguistics, who develops early-onset Alzheimer's. The book is written as if by her. Alice is fifty years old, a runner and seemingly in good health, with none of the afflictions of older people. As the disease progresses, Alice undergoes tests, has consultations with specialists, makes lists of things to do, Googles to learn more about the disease, invites others with early-onset Alzheimer's to her home and uses her Blackberry as an *aide-memoire*.

Still Alice contains insights on life in one of the intellectual powerhouses of the United States. When Alice tells her head of department that she has Alzheimer's, he seems less concerned with her condition than with a possible scandal: "Parents are paying forty grand a year. This wouldn't go over well with them." When Alice goes public, her colleagues offer condolences, but none of them sit beside her in a seminar. This kind of avoidance and stigmatization reminds me of the time I calmed down a man having a fit near our trading post in Sokoto, Nigeria. The head of our labour gang, an elderly Muslim, shook his head at me, telling me that I might have "caught" the man's condition.

Still Alice ends on a hopeful note. Her husband appears more interested in his career than in his wife's condition; he fiddles with his wedding ring whenever her health is discussed and takes a job in New York. The novel does not follow Alice into the severe stages of Alzheimer's. It ends with her holding a baby on her lap, watching her actress daughter present a monologue. She asks her mother how she feels. Alice replies, "I feel love. It's about love."

John Bayley's books on his life with his wife Iris Murdoch, once considered the most brilliant woman in Britain, present a different picture of caring for a sufferer of Alzheimer's. A novelist and philosopher, Murdoch was diagnosed with it in 1998, but appears to have developed it about five years earlier. In *Iris: A Memoir of Iris Murdoch* and *Iris and Her Friends*, Bayley, a professor of English literature at Oxford University, tells of fumbling through as his wife's dementia worsened. He did not rely on tests or expert advice as he struggled to do his best for his wife. He mentions the *solitude á deux* that marked his marriage, as it did ours: "One of the truest pleasures [of it] is solitude." Bayley and Murdoch lived alone together, as Pat and I did, moving both closer and further apart during their married life, developing in their own way while sharing mutual joys.

A movie, *Iris*, tells the story of their life before and after she developed dementia. Placed in a nursing home, Iris refused to eat or drink in the last stages of Alzheimer's, dying at seventy-nine, a year after her diagnosis.

The old cliché, if you don't use it, you lose it, does not seem to apply to the mind. Our caregivers told me that they mainly looked after "educated people," professionals who obviously once had active minds. This observation may reflect that such people have the means to pay for the services of caregivers. We paid just over $300 a month for six hours of service a week and could easily afford this.

Pat, who earned four university degrees, was a lifelong learner. In 1991, at the age of sixty-one, she noted that her memory was "declining alarmingly." Three years later, Pat worried about developing Alzheimer's. Did this become a self-fulfilling prophecy? Pat suffered from atrial fibrillation in the 1990s. No cause could be found for these rapid and irregular heartbeats, but they have been identified as one of the "putative risks" — doctors seldom talk about causes of diseases these days — associated with vascular cognitive impairment. Were Pat's fibrillations connected to her dementia? In 2004, she was diagnosed with temporal arteritis, an inflammation of the muscular walls of the scalp. She took prednisone for it, a drug that can have serious side effects, including damage to the immune system. Did this disease and its treatment bring on Pat's dementia? Pat also suffered from hypertension, the elevation of the arterial blood pressure above the normal range, once ending up in Emergency with it. This, too, has been identified as a putative risk in the genesis of dementia.

Is dementia a disease of civilization, of accelerated change, the hyperactivity of the wired world, consumerism and a society based on materialism, entitlement and discontent that generates anxiety, depression and stress? An item in the Halifax *Chronicle Herald* of October 22, 2011, claimed that experiencing depression during life can double the risk of developing Alzheimer's, and perhaps other forms of dementia, when women reach old age.

The links between stress and dementia are also being studied. With more people on earth and more people living longer, all kinds of factors can influence the incidence of dementia. People can have Alzheimer's for ten years before symptoms appear. Research on dementia reveals that it may resemble cancer in not having one single cause. And, therefore, there can be no single cure.

I did not puzzle overmuch about the causes of Pat's dementia while recognizing that it would worsen over time. I read all I could about the disease while caring for her, but did not overburden my mind with too much information on dementia. And I learned more about how memory works.

The Theft of Memory

> *Alzheimer's…is the greatest thief of memory…in*
> *terms of how much it steals and how many it steals*
> *from — both patients and caregivers.*
>
> Steve Joordens, *Memory and the Human*
> *Lifespan*

Memory is not one "thing," a single entity or presence in the brain; it has many aspects. Implicit memory records repeated experiences without any deliberate effort. Working memory, also known as short-term memory, helps us to do every-day things without thinking about them. What we learn by exercising it passes into long-term memory. It consists of semantic, procedural and episodic memory. Semantic memory is the library in our brain from which we retrieve the information we need, when we need it. Licensed cab drivers in London learn "The Knowledge," hundreds of routes, landmarks, points of interest in the city, storing this information in their semantic memory. When a fare hires a cab, the driver recalls the shortest way to his or her destination. Procedural memory, also known as muscle memory, enables the cab driver to take his vehicle through the labyrinth of London's streets, turning, stopping, starting, looking into the rearview mirror, without conscious effort. Once you learn to ride a bicycle, you never forget it — or so the story goes. With episodic memory, we recall specific events in the past as if we switched on a movie projector or put a DVD into the player.

Emotional memory, the deepest and least understood aspect, has obvious implications for those caring from sufferers from dementia. The outbursts, insults and bad language that occur from time to time may be rooted in memories of the past that you, and the sufferer, have long forgotten but that suddenly surface.

Some parts of memory are seemingly indestructible, as is some sense of personality. Even in the severe stages of dementia, Pat was always Pat to me. Her essential being remained intact, even as her responses to me changed dramatically.

A woman with dementia featured in the National Film Board documentary *Labour of Love* suddenly turns on her son and a patient in a nursing home: "Shut up. What the hell do you know? Kiss my arse." Another woman, being cared for at home by her son says to him, "You have an unhappy look on your face. What's wrong?"

If a person has been kind, well mannered and responsive before developing dementia, they will continue largely to be that way during the illness. If an individual has always been nasty before being afflicted with dementia, his or her pattern of behaviour will continue as before. As William Faulkner put it, "The past is not dead. It's not even past."

Memory harbours many mysteries. Episodic memory goes first in dementia as sufferers forget what they heard or saw a few minutes ago. And so they ask the same question again and again. The loss of short-term memory can be a blessing. The sufferer quickly forgets your bad behaviour. At times, I blew my cool, shouted at Pat, told her she was no longer the person I married. She immediately forgot my outbursts. Once, after shouting at Pat, I apologized. She said, "I don't mind." Even in the depths of dementia, Pat remained the forgiving person she had ever been.

Over the years, semantic and procedural memory fades. Dementia patients forget who they are, where they are and how to do things they have done automatically throughout their lives. This does not appear to be a linear process. Memories are not simply factual replays of past events. They are reconstructed from bits and pieces of information stored in the brain. Sufferers can have wonderful moments of lucidity and maintain their procedural memory in the last stages of dementia.

Two friends comparing notes on mothers with dementia likened the experience of caring for them to being near a lighthouse. Once in a while, their mothers would "light up" before returning to the darkness of dementia.

I compared caring for Pat to looking for a black cat in an unlighted cellar. From time to time, someone struck a match and I caught sight of it. Caring for a person with dementia resembles doing a jigsaw puzzle without the illustration and becoming aware that half the pieces are missing. On February 4, 2012, Pat told me her name, but had no idea where she was. In the last year of her life, Pat's procedural memory appeared to have vanished. She ate her food, including ice cream and trifle, with her fingers. Yet, five days before she died, Pat went to the bathroom on her own.

Alzheimer's and other dementias have three, or perhaps four, stages: mild, moderate, severe and very severe. The Global Deterioration Scale describes seven stages from the first (No decline. Experiences no problems of daily living.) to the last (Very severe cognitive decline. Becomes unable to smile.). The stages look neat on paper. However, determining when dementia begins and when sufferers move from one stage to the next represents yet another of its mysteries. In theory, each stage lasts a year to a year and a half. But there is no certainty in this. Some of those afflicted with Alzheimer's, like Iris Murdoch, die shortly after diagnosis. Others live for years, unable to speak or walk. Death usually comes from causes other than dementia. I could never tell at what stage Pat was until almost her last days; she seemed to be on a plateau during most of the years of her dementia.

Diagnosing dementia and tracing its course can be incredibly difficult, as I found while caring for Pat, and as Drs. Ken Rockwood and Chris MacKnight report in *Understanding Dementia*. And the response of families to a diagnosis can be even more baffling.

Diagnosing Dementia

*In 20 years of dementia specialist practice, I have
seen families torn apart by a dementia diagnosis. I
have also seen them come together.*

Dr. Ken Rockwood, *"Dementia will only
become more common,"* The Chronicle Herald,
October 30, 2011

Like old age, dementia creeps up on people, stealing their
minds, slowly, stealthily, inexorably. And nothing can be done
about it. Early diagnosis can help in planning the care of a
sufferer. The case studies in Rockwood and MacKnight's
Understanding Dementia reveal how difficult it can be to separate dementia from other ailments that affect the mind. These
examples read like short stories, most of which end unhappily.
They show how important the family and social context of
those stricken with dementia are in making a diagnosis. A
sixty-two-year-old woman reported memory loss and disorientation. Ruling out Alzheimer's, vascular dementia, depression
and delirium, the doctors concluded she had Creutzfeld-Jakob
disease. This was confirmed "pathologically" — by an autopsy.

Injuries may make people prone to Alzheimer's. A patient
fractured his hip, had surgery and "a sudden onset of dementia following an episode of delirium." Another case study
indicates a problem with highly educated retired people who
are no longer at the top of their game. A seventy-one-year-old
former professor, Mr. J., became concerned about his memory;
his bridge playing had deteriorated and he had difficulty reading the stock tables. He was sure that his friends were noticing
these problems. A CT scan and blood work showed nothing

abnormal. Mr. J. was diagnosed with "age associated memory impairment," a common condition of older people.

Reassured, the man left the clinic "apparently happy." He now had a name for what ailed him. Mr. J. returned nine months later, telling the doctors that "things had clearly gotten worse." Neuropsychological testing ruled out depression and anxiety. Once again, the man experienced "apparent relief." Five months later, Mr. J. was back at the clinic, "sure that things were worse."

Rockwood and MacKnight comment, "The problem is twofold; the patient has isolated, apparently non-progressive memory impairment, and he is not coping well with it." Away from students and peers, the retired professor lost the stimulus from interacting with them. He refused counseling, went back to the care of his family physician and adapted more effectively to the problems of his failing memory. Tests a few years later showed no significant changes in Mr. J.'s mind, and he "appeared less worried and continues to function well." About half the patients showing memory impairment can develop dementia within four years, but not in this case.

Rockwood and MacKnight wrote *Understanding Dementia* to assist general practitioners, family doctors and others to diagnose dementia. Doing so, they write, "can be difficult and time consuming." Primary care providers will be seeing more and more patients who may or may not have dementia, given the increased media coverage of the disease. The authors outline the most effective way to deal with those who may be suffering from dementia in five fifteen-minute visits.

The first visit seeks to answer the question, Does the patient with a memory complaint have a memory problem? The second asks, What type of memory impairment is present? Does the patient have dementia? If the patient is diagnosed with dementia, the next visit seeks to determine what kind it is and the one after that explores what can be done. On the fifth and final visit, the medical practitioner seeks to determine if the dementia is progressing as expected, whether new behavioural or medical problems have arisen and what help the caregiver needs.

From here on, the onus for caring for the sufferer is on his or her family. Although *Understanding Dementia* is written for a medical readership, its simple, plain style makes it accessible to caregivers. The book contains checklists to identify symptoms of memory loss and the general medical condition of a patient. I kept careful notes of Pat's behaviour and told the doctors what I knew of her mental and physical state. In dealing with dementia, it is vital for caregivers to keep doctors informed, to see themselves as partners during the diagnosis and the progress of the disease. They have also to recognize that, beyond a certain point, the medical profession can do nothing for sufferers unless they contract a disease or suffer an injury.

Our life would have been much easier had we to contend only with Pat's failing memory. No one gets sick or falls ill these days — they have health issues. And Pat had lots of these. During and after 2005, our life seemed to consist of an endless round of visits to doctors, clinics and pharmacies as we coped with Pat's medical problems. They included not only atrial fibrillation and hypertension, but also shingles (herpes zoster), kidney problems, osteoporosis, cataracts, anxiety and depression. Pat endured all these ailments with grace and courage, seldom complaining, seeking always to keep our life as normal as possible.

All the health professionals we encountered provided excellent care for her. And they cared about her. One thanked a colleague for the opportunity to look after this "delightful family." Our family doctor noted that Pat had "a lovely, healthy supportive husband." My health stayed excellent while I cared for Pat, save for a slight touch of cancer that put me in hospital in 2008.

Even in the depths of her dementia, Pat always thanked those who cared for her; however, not all encounters with health professionals went smoothly.

A dental technician upset Pat when she had her teeth cleaned. She was referred to the Dalhousie University Dentistry Clinic where everyone made Pat welcome in a beautiful, gleaming setting. So much at ease did Pat feel here that she once fell asleep in the chair.

The office of the ophthalmologist who looked after Pat's infected eye — she had a virus in it and macular degeneration — had the dreary ambiance of an abandoned station where old people huddled as if waiting for a train that would never come. Appointments meant nothing; we usually had to be there for an hour before being seen. On one visit, while I struggled to seat Pat in the examination chair, a staff member stood by. I said to her, angrily, "Can't you see she has dementia?" The woman replied, "That's not my specialty." She was much more helpful on our next visit.

Diagnosing Pat

> *Seventy is wormwood,*
> *Seventy is gall,*
> *But it's better to be seventy*
> *Than not alive at all.*

Phyllis McGinley, on her seventieth birthday

As the new millennium opened, Pat became increasingly worried about her memory. She acquired books, made lists and did crossword puzzles; our thesaurus fell apart from overuse. I bought a copy of *The Bantam Medical Dictionary* to learn more about Pat's ailments. I asked Pat's ophthalmologist what was wrong with her right eye. He mumbled, "Involution." Looking this up, I discovered it meant "atrophy of an organ in old age."

We were blessed with our family doctor, Deanna Swinemar, brisk, cheerful and down-to-earth. I mentioned my painful housemaid's knee, fluid accumulating in the front of the kneecap, acquired while polishing my bed spaces during my time in the Royal Air Force, to Deanna. She said, "Don't kneel."

I secured Pat's medical file after her death and traced the progress of her dementia. A report from Dr. Swinemar dated July 26, 2002, stated that Pat was "very pleasant [and] frail appearing...has always seemed to be very anxious to me since we met 4 years ago."

Deanna tested Pat with the Mini–Mental State Examination (MMSE), a game of thirty questions, on August 6, 2002. The first question is "What year is this?" Objects are named or shown ("Kim's game") and the patient asked to recall them and to count back from a hundred by sevens. Copying a clock face, a house and a polygon reveals the progress of the disease. Numbers drop off the dial, the house and the polygon become mere straggling lines over time as the dementia moves from the mild to the very severe stage. Pat scored thirty out of thirty on her first MMSE test.

On October 31, 2002, Pat went on her own to the Memory Disability Clinic. Dr. Susan Freter, a geriatrician, described her (twice) as "a lovely 72 year old lady" in her report. Pat stated that she had been having problems with her memory for five years. The doctor noted, "She complains that she is having more difficulty multitasking than usual and she thinks that she is having word-finding difficulty and short-term forgetfulness." Pat denied being depressed, adding that her anxiety had improved considerably. She was concerned about developing dementia as a number of her friends had it; this was news to me for I knew none of them so afflicted. Dr. Freter stated that I was not concerned about Pat's memory loss, nor were any of her friends. Her report concluded, "Mrs. Lotz is quite highly functioning and is independent in her way of living, as well as her instrumental activities of daily living...there is no evidence of any objective cognitive deficit." One of Dr. Freter's comments echoed the report in *Understanding Dementia* about Mr. J. Pat was experiencing minor changes associated with aging: "...as a highly functioning intelligent woman, she may be more introspective and putting more weight on normal occurrences than they are due."

Is the higher incidence of dementia among women due to their fear of aging as they are constantly bombarded by messages from advertisers and the media about the need to be and to look forever young? Another mystery among many about dementia.

Pat's stubborn nature and dislike of medication emerges in a report by Dr. Virginia Walford, a psychologist she consulted in 2002 to help her cope with our daughter Annette's death and the guilt she felt about not being present at it. Dr. Welford reported that Pat was adamant in refusing medication for what she diagnosed as depression for fear of side effects and addiction: "Patricia is an independent and intelligent woman [who has] difficulty in asking for and receiving help…" Pat at one time took Zoloft, but quit using this.

Our life went on normally for a couple of years.

Orthotics resolved a problem Pat had with her feet; increased fluid intake took care of a kidney complaint. The temporal arteritis that she contracted in April 2004 eventually cleared up with prednisone, a corticosteroid, which thinned her hair. That obviously damaged her morale. Pat's hair eventually came back, more beautiful than ever.

On August 11, 2004, Pat saw Dr. Caroline Abbott, who described her as "frail, well groomed and well dressed… calm and able to smile occasionally." She added, "She is very tired, she has gone from being an active person to needing support to walk. She feels very dependent. She says she has 'lost contact with myself.' I believe she means her cognitive ability has changed from someone with a lot going on in her thinking and feeling to someone who has very little going on and has difficulty expressing her thoughts. She is a writer with a sharp intellect and used to read a lot and now is no longer able to express that. There is a lack of enjoyment and an anxiety about her condition and she has had significant weight loss."

Dr. Abbott checked her memory, concluding that Pat had "a fairly rapid deterioration in intellectual ability and memory…with the family history of Alzheimer's Disease this is the first thing that comes to mind."

Pat was always resistant to medication, and I wondered if those she was taking were having adverse side effects.

On August 13, 2004, Pat and I went to the Memory Disability Clinic and met with Dr. Laurie Mallery, a geriatrician. I told her that Pat awoke each morning with great fear, had become weak, was feeling unwell and had little appetite.

Pat scored twenty-six out of thirty on the MMSE but showed signs of memory impairment. Her severe depression and anxiety made it difficult to assess her cognition.

Towards the end of 2004, Pat developed herpes. If you have chickenpox as a child, the virus stays in your body, causing herpes if the immune system falters. Did the drugs that Pat took weaken hers? Pat developed a rash on her upper body, and we lost one of the greatest joys of married life, cuddling in bed, content and at peace in each other's arms. We could no longer do this for the rash was painful for Pat. We resorted to just holding hands, which is not quite the same thing as cuddling… Postherpetic pain followed the outbreak of shingles.

At first, I was angry at Pat becoming ill, thinking only of my own needs and of what I would be deprived. This feeling soon passed, especially as I saw how well she handled the pain from shingles. I became Pat's medication manager, ensuring she took her pills and putting drops in her eyes. She appreciated this at first, but giving Pat her meds would become increasingly difficult. I made up supermilk and gave her Ensure to help her put on weight.

On October 6, 2005, Pat returned to the Memory Clinic on her own. By this time she cooked only one meal a week and we relied on Meals on Wheels for the rest of the time. Pat told Dr. Mallery that she was losing her train of thought and forgetting what I told her. She scored twenty-seven out of thirty on the MMSE, but her clock drawing was asymmetrical and abnormal and she had no recollection of current events. Dr. Mallery concluded that Pat did not meet the criteria for dementia and had no "functional impairment."

Pat and I returned to the Memory Clinic on October 19. She could no longer remember the names of our children and had difficulty recalling those of her siblings and the titles of the three books she was reading. I suggested to Dr. Mallery that some of Pat's problems might stem from her medications. She suggested reducing the gabapentin Pat was taking for postherpetic pain; its side effects include dizziness, sedation, fatigue and constipation. I also reduced Pat's intake of prednisone.

I noted in my diary on November 25, 2005, "I feel I can do so little for her." Throughout the time of Pat's dementia, I had a continual struggle as a caregiver. How much should I do for Pat, and how much could she do for herself? I wanted her to retain as much as possible of her autonomy and independence. Pat's self-reliance had always been important to me, as mine had been to her.

A CT scan on May 21, 2006, showed increased cerebral atrophy, a common feature of the brains of older people. But "no acute process intercranially," which presumably meant an absence of the tangles and clumps of Alzheimer's.

Despite Pat's memory problems and her ailments, our life proceeded tranquilly and serenely as I adapted to my role as her caregiver. Pat cooked meals, cleaned the house, sorted through files and clothing, throwing away what she no longer needed, made lists and kept a calendar to remember dates.

On August 10, 2006, we returned to the Memory Clinic and saw Dr. Paige King. Pat scored twenty-one out of thirty on the Montreal Cognitive Assessment. Dr. Paige noted that Pat's "verbal fluency was intact and clock drawing test abnormal." She asked Pat if she could plan a dinner party for twelve people. She said she could. Dr. Paige wrote, "Mrs. Lotz has a lifelong history of being a worrier… She says her mood is perhaps more low than it has been previously, although she continues to enjoy activities. She feels that if there is no change in her health, the future looks dreary." She added, "Mental status exam today revealed a woman who was well kept... There was normal thought content and process." The diagnosis: cognitive impairment: no dementia (CIND).

If I had to put a date on the time when Pat's forgetfulness turned into dementia, it would probably be the fall of 2006. On June 23, 2007, I wrote to Dr. Swinemar about Pat's mental deterioration before Christmas in the previous year. I listed my observations:

Pat had no short-term memory and kept asking me the same questions.

She was confused and anxious and kept losing things.

She saw and heard people, some of whom she claimed were taking her clothes.

She once read a book or two each week. Now she reads and rereads the same book, unaware that she is doing so.

She had stopped cooking meals.

At Christmas, we always watched her favourite movies, *The Holly and the Ivy*, *A Christmas Carol* (with Alistair Sim) and *A Child's Christmas in Wales*. She showed no interest in viewing them, nor in receiving a large number of small presents from me, another Christmas ritual.

At times she did not know who I was.

I added, "Pat remains as loving and lovable as ever, and has retained her sense of humour. At least she still laughs at my jokes!"

On August 2, 2007, we went again to the Memory Clinic. Despite her confusion, Pat still chose her own clothing and continued to be well dressed and well groomed. Dr. Mallery reported, "Mr. Lotz has had trouble understanding the cause of [his wife's strange] behaviors. He describes that he is generally patient; however, on 3 occasions, he lost his temper and yelled at his wife."

She scored twenty-four out of thirty on the MMSE, but her clock drawing was "very abnormal." She knew the name of the president of the United States but not that of her father.

Dr. Mallery concluded, "In summary, Mrs. Lotz has had cognitive impairment since 2004, which has slowly been progressing over time, with a possible more rapid decline in December 2006." Her examination revealed "impairment of memory and executive function...consistent with a diagnosis of Alzheimer disease and possible vascular dementia, of moderate stage."

I had no inkling before the fall of 2006 that Pat was developing dementia. I thought she was just having the usual problems with her memory as old people do. I began to see that most of our problems arose from my stupidity and lack of understanding, not from Pat's behaviour.

Somehow we had gone through the early onset of Alzheimer's without recognizing it. I failed to ask Dr. Mallery for a letter that I could have used for a disability claim on Pat's income tax.

I told Dr. Mallery I did not want Pat told of the diagnosis, and we discussed the use of Aricept, which slows down dementia. With Pat's atrial flutter and weight loss (for which no cause could be found) "it was felt that the risk of the medication outweighed the benefits."

Our life entered a different phase.

The strain of caring for Pat began to wear me down, and I decided to go to Britain in October 2007, to do research. Pat's sister Marie agreed to look after her but had difficulty doing so. On a day of pouring rain, Pat put on her coat and told Marie, "This is not my home." She headed for the door. Marie tried to restrain her. Pat grew angry and threw a plaque through a side window of the front door and headed for the street. In one of the many acts of kindness we experienced, some young men passing Thorndean recognized Pat's condition. They walked her around the block, calming her down, and took her back home. A friend found matching glass for the broken window and replaced it at no cost.

Wandering is a feature of dementia sufferers. But it's not an irrational act. Pat obviously wanted to get away from her sister even if it meant leaving the house in pouring rain. Only once while I was caring for her did Pat wander away from Thorndean, the house she loved.

At times, Pat was quite lucid, at other times confused, starting but not ending sentences, another feature of dementia. She was afraid of what might come from outside the house, insisting that the door be always locked and the drapes drawn.

In November 2007, I wrote in my diary, "The confusion continues. This morning Pat took towels out of the cupboard, thinking they needed to be washed. She has mislaid both her pairs of glasses, and for the last three nights has slept in her clothes, taking off only her slacks. She continually says 'You know' and 'Oh, dear.'"

I recognize now that these expressions reflected her increasing confusion and loss. Since Pat died, I've been saying "Oh, dear" a lot.

As Pat's condition worsened and she relied more and more on me to do daily tasks, I wrote in my diary, "It's as if part of me encloses Pat, cares for her, looks after her needs, loves her. While another bit switches on when needed, giving me time and space to do what I want to do. So there is some balance in my life."

Pat had a plate in her mouth to replace two missing front teeth — and lost it. And the replacement. Again and again, she asked me what she could do for me, talked about going back to Britain, said she wanted to go home to see her mother and burst into tears when I told her she was seventy-seven. She also asked me why her father did not come to see her. I made the mistake of telling Pat that he was dead, which upset her. Later I would say that he was busy or back in Britain. She suddenly asked me when Dino would come in and was surprised when I told her that he was "no longer with us."

Most of the time, life went on without too many upsets, until the summer of 2008, when I was diagnosed with cancer of the cecum, a part of my body I never knew I had. It lies at the junction of the small and large intestine. Like the appendix, it appears to have no function except to become diseased. In late September, I went into hospital to have my cecum removed with laparoscopic surgery. I had excellent care. Dr. Paul Johnson, the surgeon, seemed more worried about the cancer than I was. I was damned if I'd let a little thing like that stop me from caring for Pat.

I went into hospital on a Monday in September 2008 and left on the following Friday, immediately setting off to recover Pat from the Berkeley, a posh residence, where she had spent the week. The staff had not been too pleased with her. Several times she had escaped, walking on one occasion for two kilometres before being found. If proof is needed that the best place for people with dementia is the home, Pat's perambulations while I was in hospital offer abundant proof.

And so we again picked up our normal routine. With our experience of what happened when I was in hospital, I wrote on May 29, 2009, to Dr. Swinemar, asking for a geriatric assessment in case I proved unable to care for Pat. I ended the letter, "Some days, some hours, are better than others, but I expect this is the pattern for most caregiver–care receiver relationships."

On October 15, we went again to the Memory Disability Clinic and saw Dr. Mallery. She had launched the PATH (Palliative and Therapeutic Harmonization) programme. This initiative illustrates Jung's axiom "Only the wounded physician can heal." Dr. Mallery, with the help of her mother and sister, removed her father from a hospital so he could spend his last days in comfort and peace in his own home. She tells how hospitals and the medical profession in the United States hold on to patients as a way of maintaining cash flow in her amusing book *The Salami Salesman and his Daughter Falafel*. PATH recognizes the unpleasant truth about old age: It ends in death. And for many seniors, little can be done to cure their ailments. The PATH handbook states, "While the medical treatment of frail elderly individuals can result in desirable outcomes, indiscriminate use of aggressive interventions at the end of life can cause paradoxical harm and suffering."

I was grateful for the straightforward way in which Dr. Mallery spoke to me about Pat's condition. As the dementia progressed, communication became more difficult. I thought Pat's hearing was failing. Dr. Mallery assured me this was not the problem; Pat's brain was having increasing difficulty in deciphering what I was saying.

On our visit, Dr. Mallery reviewed Pat's medical history, noting that "She is a highly intelligent woman." Pat scored only nine out of thirty on the MMSE, could not remember my name or that of our daughters and did badly on the clock test. She still had neuropathic pain from the shingles and had developed kyphosis, also known as widow's hump, a spinal curvature caused by the way she hunched her back.

Dr. Mallery told me, "This is the best she will ever be," and gave me a letter stating that Pat had "severe (end-stage) Alzheimer dementia. She requires total care for Activities of Daily Living and constant 24-hour, supervision." This letter secured a disability benefit on Pat's income tax.

After this session, I wrote in my diary, "We've had a good life together, so must make the best of these, our last days." I recognized that our life had entered a new phase and that I had to have help in caring for Pat. Norma Minard of the Provincial Continuing Care Department came to our home to discuss the options. It would take about three months of paperwork and procedures if I wanted to put Pat into a nursing home. I was eligible for ten hours a week of respite and sixty days a year of care in a nursing home at a subsidized rate. I decided to take six hours of respite a week. Despite the difficulties of caring for Pat, I still enjoyed her company and looked forward to seeing her on my return from respite on Wednesday and Saturday afternoons.

At the end of October 2009, I went on my own to see Dr. Mallery. She wrote, "Mr. Lotz indicates that care was a burden at times, but that his wife, overall, was easy to take care of. He feels committed to her care and does not find it excessively onerous. He says he tries to control his own attitude and cherishes the moments they have together. He views the persistent care of his wife as a commitment to his marriage vows."

My role as a carer went beyond that. It was rooted in the deep, passionate, enduring love I had for Pat. Dr. Mallery described the adverse effects that medical interventions might cause: "Mrs. Lotz would be considered to be in the final phase of her life...and decisions should be made based on that determination."

I returned for a final session with Dr. Mallery on October 29, 2009.

I had medical consent, a legal document that appointed me as Pat's guardian "to consent or refuse medical treatment or give directions respecting medical treatment at any time in the future when I am no longer capable of directing my medical treatment." With Dr. Mallery's help, I worked out a plan to care for Pat. I stated that I did not want resuscitation, surgery or complex treatments (radiation, chemotherapy) for her, but she should receive antibiotics if she had a severe disease. I wanted Pat to be treated at home but would prefer her to die in hospital. On Dr. Mallery's advice, I stopped giving Pat Zoloft, but continued with the beta blocker (for her atrial fibrillation), warfarin (a blood thinner) and Xylocaine, an ointment for neuropathic pain. Dr. Mallery suggested stopping the Alendronate for osteoporosis and I eventually did this. Giving Pat pills and eye drops had become burdensome.

Dr. Mallery's report concluded with a note on symptom management: "Mr. Lotz felt that multiple medications had been tried in the past for improved control of the herpes zoster and neck pain. He felt that the adverse effects of these medications were worse than the symptoms themselves and...he was not interested in trying additional medication."

The authors of *Understanding Dementia* pose a question about those diagnosed with dementia: "Is treatment of this condition now likely to do more harm than good?"

Woody Allen once stated that he didn't mind dying, he just did not want to be there when it happened. The PATH programme forces caregivers to face tough decisions as those they love enter the last days of their life. They can panic or do nothing or decide to manage their lives and those for whom they care to ensure as good a quality of life as possible as the loved one becomes frailer and frailer.

This is what I tried to do.

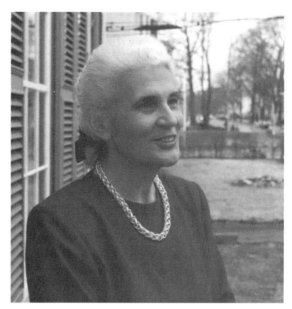

Pat grown lovelier with age, outside
Thorndean, 1993.

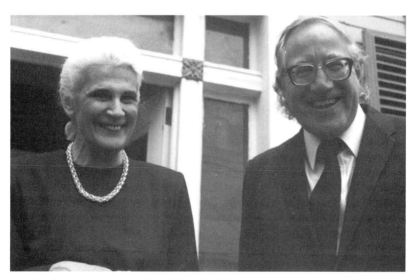

Pat and Jim at the entrance to Thorndean.

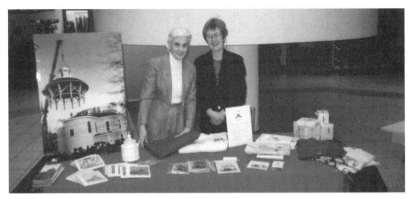

Pat and Anne West at St. George's Church restoration exhibit, City Centre Atlantic's Heritage Expo, 1996.

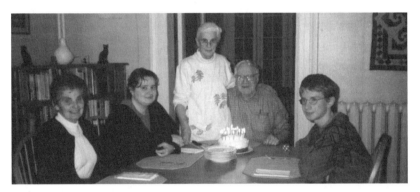

Celebrating Pat's sixty-ninth birthday at Thorndean in October 1999. From the left, Pat's sister Marie, daughter Fiona, Pat, Jim and grandson Peter.

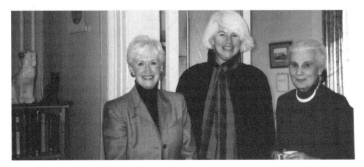

Guests Leila Gashus and Jill Robinson with Pat at the All Broads' Lunch, August 2000.

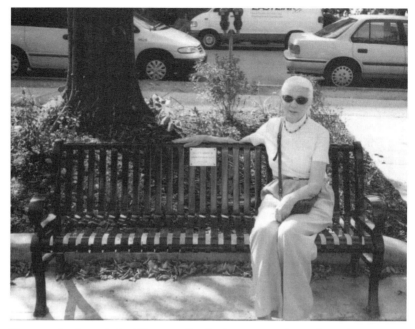

Pat on the bench in Victoria Park that we endowed in the memory of our daughter Annette, summer 2003.

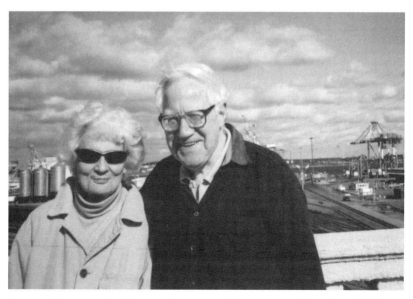

Pat and Jim on the Young Avenue rail overpass, October 2007.

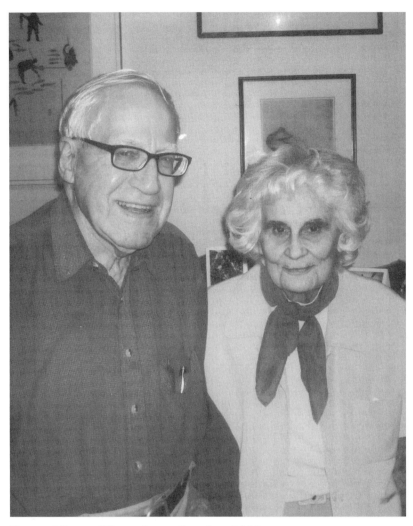

Jim and Pat at Thorndean, October 2009.

Chapter Seven
Managing Dementia: Never a Dull Moment

Where I am, I don't know, I'll never know, in the silence you don't know, you must go on, I can't go on, I'll go on.

Samuel Beckett, *The Unnamable*

The words of the enigmatic Irish writer catch the essence of life with a person with dementia. As Pat's main caregiver, I learned to be a detached observer and a sensitive responder to her needs. At first I denied that Pat had dementia and became impatient with the way she behaved. When she was diagnosed with cognitive impairment, I recognized that she would eventually succumb to dementia.

To me, as to many others, the diagnosis of Alzheimer's came as something of a relief. I knew now that Pat would never get better, that she would slowly but surely drift away from me. I had to hope for the best and prepare for the worst. If you learn how to manage a loved one's dementia, you can have a rich and rewarding — and interesting — life together.

When dementia strikes, it's natural to focus on what is being lost: memory, attention, customary rituals, routines, regularities, reciprocities and responses. The person with dementia is still a human being who needs love, support and acceptance, no matter how bizarre his or her behaviour. You have to continually seek what remains of the person you love, to find vital sparks and do your best to fan them into flame.

Our lives did not suddenly change when Pat was diagnosed with Alzheimer's. We kept to our usual routines, and I did all I could to ensure Pat's happiness. Before the diagnosis, in February 2008, I wrote in my diary, "Actually, all in all, I remain surprised at how normal things are, despite Pat's absence of short-term memory. I do what I can to help her, but lose my patience from time to time. Keeping a balance, keeping Pat happy has become a major undertaking these days. I tell her to make the most of small joys, take each day at a time and concentrate on getting through it."

In July 2008, our daughter Fiona moved to Victoria where she remarried. Our grandson Peter stayed in Halifax and became a granny sitter from time to time.

Pat's behaviour became odder and odder as the dementia progressed. She saw people in the front garden, a shrub becoming a crouching man. Pat cried when she thought that her sister Marie had died, talked about going to Thorndean, asked me if I had a car and looked for another Jim in her life. Pat wanted to go into hospital and to find work, telling me that she thought she was living in a fairy tale. She continually spoke of "going home" — a common phenomenon of dementia sufferers — of returning to England. People kept stealing her stuff, including two sweaters that I'd found she'd put in a bag.

From time to time, even deep in dementia, Pat would have moments of normality and lucidity. She once said, "It's not fair to you, looking after me." I told her, "Fairness has nothing to do with it. I do what I do because I love you."

Pat kept her sense of humour, and this helped to sustain me. A friend gave us a fruitcake. I offered a slice to Pat, saying, "It's very rich. But we can afford it." And she smiled. If a show on TV showed the Sistine Chapel or the walls of a European palace, I'd joke, "You can't get wallpaper like that these days." Pat would laugh.

Asleep, she looked as serene and beautiful as ever. Gazing at her, a corny 1970s song came to mind, something about "just watching you sleep, my heart overflowing with love." Pat remained self-reliant even as the dementia eroded her mind. I would leave her on her own to go to the library or to do the groceries, never worrying she would get into trouble. On April 23, 2008, we had lunch out for the first time in a year — and the last. Before leaving the house, Pat made sure her lipstick was on straight.

Pat moved into an Alice in Wonderland world as her life became "curiouser and curiouser."

She no longer knew who she was and who these strangers, including me, were. And I had to believe six impossible things about her before breakfast.

In November 2009, when the first home support worker arrived, I had a tremendous sense of relief and freedom as I left the house for three hours during which I could do as I pleased.

I took a respite month in April 2010 while Pat lived in a nursing home. I checked it beforehand, finding it clean and obviously well run. I did not tell Pat she was leaving home and going into care.

When I took Pat to her room in the nursing home, she thought I would be staying there with her. The dismay and anguish in Pat's eyes as I kissed her goodbye haunt me still. In the note I sent to the nursing home with her list of medications, I wrote, "Despite her dementia, Pat is a wonderful person whose kindness surfaces from time to time. But she needs more care than I can give her." I noticed that the staff of the home avoided my gaze as I left Pat in her room. Outside the place, I felt that I had my life back again. I phoned once to determine how Pat was doing, having decided that I would not visit her in the home. She was causing no problems, wandering around in her dressing gown and eating well. I wondered whether the time had come to put Pat into care.

I first flew to New York to take part in a PBS "American Experience" programme on the 1881–1884 Greely expedition to Northern Ellesmere Island. Returning to Halifax, I travelled to Kitchener for the release of a reprint of my book *Understanding Canada*, originally published in 1977, and on to Victoria to visit our daughter and do research.

Refreshed by the respite, I wrote in my diary before setting out to bring Pat home, "Whatever the frustrations, life is better with Pat than without her. She provides a great deal of stimulation…"

I was shocked when I saw Pat. Looking frailer than ever, her lovely hair uncombed and in a mess, so diminished had she become during our time apart that I almost did not recognize her. Her beautiful eyes lit up when she saw me. We hugged each other while waiting for the taxi to take us home. Here I held her close with tears in my eyes, writing later, "I'll do all I can to avoid putting Pat in a home. She is sleeping now and is safe with me. I only hope she knows that, and that I adore her as I always have." We had a couple of difficult days while Pat settled back into our routine. I felt my heart break watching her relearning her way around our home but perked up when she called me a bastard because I wasn't "looking after the children." On the following morning, as Pat got out of bed, she said, "I do love you." And we had a very good day.

In June 2010, Pat and I took part in a documentary, *Fighting for a Good Death*, on the PATH programme. It dealt with how to make the best decisions about those nearing the end of their lives and profiled four cases from PATH. The shots of Pat and I show her looking quite frail but functioning well and me looking uncommonly cheerful. We still did the groceries together and went for walks round the block. Pat went to the bathroom on her own and retained her sense of style, noting that the red T-shirt and yellow sweater she wore did not go together. She knew my name but was convinced there was another Jim somewhere around.

I coped reasonably well with Pat as she became frailer and frailer. I recognized that my emotional state had much to do with the way Pat behaved.

And three books helped.

Oliver Sacks' *The Man Who Mistook His Wife for a Hat*, with its warm humanism, taught me to understand that people with mental problems retain, in many ways, their essential identity.

Robert Lindner's *The Fifty-Minute Hour* tells of some of the psychiatrist's cases. One concerned a man who claimed that he travelled in space and produced charts to prove it.

Instead of dismissing them as fantasies of a troubled mind, Lindner studied them carefully, entered into the man's mental world and discovered illogicalities in them, pointing out the impossibility of travelling from one point in space to another in the time the man claimed. The patient recognized that he had been living in an imaginary world and was apparently cured of his delusions. I continually sought what was rational and logical in Pat's behaviour rather than focusing on what upset me when she did something odd or unsettling.

Contented Dementia by Oliver James tells how Peggy Garner, an English housewife, developed SPECAL (Specialized Early Care for Alzheimer's) after her mother became afflicted. He writes, "Life with [her] was often like living in Alice's Wonderland." Garner put her mother into a home whose matron was interested in only two things: Could she afford the fees and was she continent. After three days, the matron called Garner, demanding that she remove her mother because she was a "wanderer."

Garner found another home, a large country house with bits added on to it and an atmosphere "reminiscent of Fawlty Towers." Run by an eccentric character known as "The Professor" from a tiny office, the place had a free and easy ambiance. The residents could do anything they liked, and after seventy-two hours "no one was ever a problem again."

SPECAL promotes unconditional acceptance of dementia sufferers and has three basic principles:

1. Don't ask questions.
2. Learn from them as the experts on their disability.

3. Always agree with everything they say, never interrupting them.

On December 31, 2010, *The New York Times* ran an article datelined Phoenix, Arizona, headed: "Giving Alzheimer's Patients Their Way, Even Chocolate." It began with the story of an afflicted ninety-six-year old woman who was "to put it mildly, a difficult case." Angry, refusing to eat, she hit staff and patients at nursing homes, leading to her ejection from them. Then she entered Beatitudes nursing home and her behaviour changed.

The article does not comment on the name of the place.

Beatitudes are blessings. The word is used to describe Christ's Sermon on the Mount (Matthew, 5:7). In it, he reversed the usual order and values of society: "Blessed are the gentle [meek, humble] for they shall inherit the earth."

The staff at Beatitudes turned the usual way of dealing with people with dementia upside down. Patients could eat anything they liked, including unlimited chocolate, sleep, bathe and dine when they wanted. The difficult woman, who loved chocolate, calmed down. Given a doll, she rocked, caressed and fed her "baby" before she ate. As the home's research director put it, "Whatever your vice, we're your folks." Anything that gives residents comfort, including a "nip" at bedtime, is permitted. The state tried to stop the home putting chocolate on the nursing chart because it was not a medication. But it proved more effective (and cheaper) in keeping residents happy than sedatives, antidepressants, potions and pills.

People with dementia are a lot saner than we think.

The article notes something that became obvious to me in caring for Pat: "Research suggests that creating positive emotional experiences...diminishes distress and behavior problems." Those with dementia have memories of old joys and good times that can be awakened. Scientists have dismissed learned practice in caring as subjective and ad hoc. As a caregiver, you operate in a subjective, ad hoc world as you struggle to make sense of what the sufferer needs, what he or she is struggling to communicate. You discover what works for them, and for you, by trial and error, through love and compassion, not scientific analysis.

Through 2010, I found it increasingly difficult to care for Pat. She looked to me for direction, then suddenly spat out hatred and anger and refused to take her pills. Once I forced them into her mouth and she screamed. I explained what might happen if she did not take her medications. This, of course, meant nothing to her. I decided it was time Pat went into a home and made, as I noted in my diary, "the hardest decision in my life."

It was Pat's reluctance to take her pills that did this. Here I was, her loving husband, doing all I could to keep her healthy and she was rejecting my best efforts! In the severe stages of dementia, small things can have catastrophic results, and I decided I could no longer care for Pat. She would have to go into a home. So I phoned Norma Minard at Continuing Care and asked her to send me the appropriate forms.

Two things happened that made me reverse my decision.

I learned that it would take several months to complete the paperwork and a year to find a place for Pat in a home, which might not necessarily be in the Halifax region. On October 5, 2010, Pat went to the bathroom and returned to the bedroom to tell me she had not flushed the toilet. I took care of this. Pat thanked me and asked if I was coming back to bed. I told her I loved her and we kissed. For one fleeting moment we recovered the sense of oneness that had been the essence of our life before Pat developed dementia. That wonderful moment strengthened my resolve to keep on caring for Pat, to give her unconditional love as I had always done. I solved the pill problem by crushing them and putting them in her food.

Hard Truths

Those afflicted with dementia will never get better, only worse, as the disease progresses. I learned to live in the immediate present and to recall memories of the past while caring for Pat. There is no way of knowing how fast or slow the dementia will proceed and no point in thinking too far into the unknowable future. As I learned, the only predictable thing about dementia is unpredictability, the only certainty, uncertainty. I never had any clues on how long Pat would live or when her dementia would suddenly become worse and I would be unable to care for her.

There's no point in waiting for Godot, for a miraculous cure, a sudden breakthrough that will bring a loved person back to you as once she or he was. A friend whose wife has dementia tracks research on it, some of which involves mice. Exactly what mice have to remember — that wonderful piece of gourmet cheese? — is a mystery to me. As he put it, "It will be too late for us if they find a cure."

But a great deal can be done to make the lives of sufferers comfortable and happy, and that is where the emphasis at present lies in the expanding field of dementia.

Boredom can be a problem, for you and the sufferer. Pat wanted to help me, to do things for me. She had made us a comfortable home, but we had never been house-proud, bent on keeping it in immaculate condition. Pat washed and dried the dishes and dusted shelves once in a while. I was not very imaginative in finding things for her to do.

Cognitive therapies based on music, art, crafts and story-telling can have some remarkable responses from those with dementia.

Fear, anger, worry, anxiety and other negative emotions make rational decision making difficult in caregiving. I discovered, at times, what a nasty person I was. I realized how much the tone of my voice and my body language influenced the way Pat behaved. People with dementia may be losing their minds, but they retain their emotions. When bad moods settled on me — and you can't avoid them — I shouted at Pat, grabbed her and upset her. As she lacked short-term memory, she almost immediately forgot my bad behaviour. But I did not and tried to keep my negative emotions under control.

The behaviour of those with dementia can change quite suddenly. Pat stopped cooking and taking her early-morning bath as the dementia became more severe, and she refused to change her clothes. She usually remained quite fragrant, although she smelled awful once in a while. I did not force her to wash or change.

I continually felt that I was not doing enough for Pat, although she never complained.

On October 16, 2010, I wrote, "I feel I should, could, love Pat more as the shadow falls over my life at the thought of losing her. It engulfs me, brings me close to tears. The image of a heavy heart is no cliché. Mine feels at times as if it is about to fall out of my chest."

Sufferers may become apathetic, anxious, irritable, aggressive, abusive, run through the gamut of emotions from laughter to tears in a matter of minutes as I saw Pat do. You have to learn to cope with Jekyll and Hyde behaviour, which I found impossible to predict.

Pat was never physically abusive, but she certainly lashed out at me verbally. She called me a "repulsive, dirty little swine," not her usual way of addressing me. She called me kind, and then, a few minutes later I was a "bastard." I laughed, saying, "So I'm a kind bastard. It's not easy being one of those. Takes years of training." Pat had a lot of anger in her when we married. It faded away during our years together, only to reemerge as her dementia worsened.

From time to time, we reached a plateau when life became quite normal for a few days. I wrote, on July 2, 2011, "Pat has been good this past week, no crises, arguments, upsets. Swayed to the music of *Coppelia* and said she liked a piece on Radio-Canada."

Hallucinations can plague people with dementia. Pat continually saw a woman in the house and I wondered if she thought this was a guardian angel. She did not seem threatened by her presence nor pleased by it.

Wandering is often a problem with sufferers from dementia. It may be a response to threatening or uncomfortable situations. Nursing homes in Germany put mock bus stops outside their doors. Residents wait there for busses that never come, become fed up and return to the home. Because Pat loved Thorndean so much she seldom wanted to stray from it and wandering never became a problem.

Pat, like other dementia sufferers, became a compulsive rearranger. She had an unerring instinct for playing around with stuff important to me. Pat moved the papers on my desk, messed with the clothing in my chest of drawers and fiddled with pill boxes. This sent me up the wall, especially when she hid my stuff. Was this behaviour a way of catching my attention? I soon learned that the apple never fell far from the tree. I developed a flair for finding lost stuff.

Of other things that vanished, I joked, "They'll find them when they pull down Thorndean in a couple of hundred years' time." I made sure that important items were not left around. A friend bought a device that allowed his wife to lower herself into the bath. It required a charger to operate it. This suddenly disappeared. As my friend put it, "She thinks she's looking after me." I had the same sense with Pat. Are compulsive actions a way for sufferers to exercise some control over their lives? Pat would pick up and carry around a book, a magazine, a DVD or some other item that seemed to comfort her. They were *hers*!

In the severe stage of dementia, sufferers may revert to childish behaviour, a fact I failed to recognize. Once, when shaving, I saw Pat coming too close and warned her off. She spat out, "I'll never come near you again." Pat tried to please me by offering me a book. If I rejected it, she threw it on the floor. Such incidents were few and far between.

Conversations became very strange. Pat started sentences in the middle and did not end them. Out of the blue, she said, "She's only part time." Talking to a small teddy bear, she told it, "Better keep my mouth shut." After I came into the living room where she had spent the night in her chair, we had the following conversation:

"Who are you?"

"I'm Jim, your husband."

"Don't be silly."

Some of the talk can be quite logical in a weird sort of way. Michael Caine's mum had dementia. He invited her to a party at his new house. She thought she was in a pub and asked her son if he was short of money. "Why do you think that?" Caine replied. His mother pointed to Shakira, Caine's wife, serving drinks and refilling glasses. "Why's she working as a barmaid?" As Caine put it, he gave up, explaining, "It's only a part-time job."

You have to enter the world of the sufferer from dementia, try to make sense of it and always respond to what she or he says. When Pat spoke, I'd reply, "I don't know about that" or "That's the way things are" or "We can't do anything about that." I was stuck for reply when, while watching a western on TV, Pat asked, "Where are my sausages?"

We had some memorable and amusing exchanges. Lying in bed, I told Pat, "You've lost your mind." She looked under the bed and said, "Maybe it's there." She kept talking while I tried to sleep and I asked her to stop. She said, "That makes sense."

A Canadian Press story, datelined January 2, 2013, dealt with a common reaction to people with dementia: stigmatization and avoidance. Headed "'See me, not my disease,' say those stigmatized because of dementia diagnosis," it told of a woman outraged when learning she had Alzheimer's. She was even more upset by the reaction to the diagnosis by those she considered her friends. One said, "Well why bother talking to someone who has Alzheimer's. They're not going to remember anyway." At the time the story appeared, the woman with Alzheimer's had not seen her "friend" for four years. Others dismissed the diagnosis: "Oh, I forget things too. You're okay."

People with dementia are not okay and need friendship and companionship more than ever. Pat and I, as writers and editors, belonged to a solitary breed of people. Our lifestyle, always friendly to all, but not particularly sociable, made us very close. People recognized that I was doing my best to care for Pat and largely left me to it. I never resented this. Two friends came to our home, gave us a splendid lunch, said they would do it again. This did not happen. My best friend, after Pat, moved to Regina while I was looking after her. Anne West, Pat's special friend, the most Christian person I have ever met, dropped by regularly with treats and her dog. Sally became a therapy dog, nuzzling up to Pat and comforting her. Roma Arsenault, who worked with Pat at *Atlantic Insight*, came by when she was in town, bringing food and checking our plants.

We received many small kindnesses from strangers. People opened doors and smiled on us. A clerk in a local post office pointed out to me that Pat's shoelaces had become undone. Pat wandered down the street and sat on the wall of a boarding house. I followed her, but did not insist she return home. A scruffy-looking bloke came out of the house and we started chatting. He told me that his wife, presumably suffering from agoraphobia, had not left their house in eight years. He asked Pat if she would like a popsicle, and when she nodded, dashed into the house and brought her one.

While clearing the front garden, I saw a stranger stop and look at the house. We began talking about Thorndean and its history. Dr. Michael Ojolecks, a dentist from Cape Breton, became a valued friend, delivering boxes of goodies that included some of his wife Etel's delicious, homemade items. Barbara Watt, a long-time friend, also brought us goodies she made.

Dementia sufferers may be more aware of what is happening to them than we realize. There is still something there in their minds. Pat's was still working, in a hit-and-miss fashion, as she struggled to make sense of the world. Much of her talk was unintelligible, especially in her last year. But flashes of it convinced me that she still had some grasp of reality, knew what was happening to her, when she said,

"I haven't any purpose."

"I can't think what I think how I think of myself."

"I can't think who I am."

"It's as if life has stopped."

"I don't know who I am."

"I want to be me."

"I have nothing."

"I feel empty."

Plans, Strategies and Tactics

The Alzheimer Society publishes useful material for caregivers. It covers ways of communicating ("Speak to the person as an adult"), describes 101 things to do with someone with Alzheimer's ("Cut out pictures from magazines") and tells how to interact with a sufferer ("Stay relaxed. Feel secure.")

The only thing you can control in caring for a person with dementia is your attitude to that person, to yourself and to life in general. And this is the result of lifelong experience. I always treated Pat as an autonomous person during the time of her dementia, as I had done throughout our married life. I never felt any desire to "possess" Pat. I suggested that she join the gym where I worked out. She showed no interest in doing so, although she did acquire an exercycle for a few years. It was always important to me that Pat be wrong in her own way, rather than right in mine. This attitude helped my efforts to care for her, although I was pushed to my limits at times.

It is essential to have a plan, strategies and tactics in caring for a person with dementia. While you live on a day-by-day basis, you have to go beyond making things up as you go along. The plan I drew up to care for Pat owed much to my experiences in community organization and development. I carried it in my head rather than writing it down.

The goals of the plan included keeping our lives as normal as possible for as long as possible, ensuring that Pat remained in our home for as long as possible, safe, content and comfortable and caring for myself so I could care for Pat.

The first step in the plan involved identifying our assets and determining the best use of them in meeting the goals. Some assets were obvious. They included our strong love for each other, Pat's kind and forgiving nature, my (usual) cheerfulness and optimism and my belief in my luck. My father claimed that if I fell into a toilet (he used a less elegant word), I would come up clutching a gold watch.

My good health and strong physique helped in caring for Pat. While a teenager in Scotland I had worked on a truck, humping bags of grain, fertilizer and coal, building my upper-body strength.

We had no financial worries, thanks to our frugal lifestyle and Pat's excellent house buying and keeping. With our condo unit on one floor, Pat did not have to ascend stairs. We lived in a quiet, friendly neighbourhood, with all medical services within a ten-dollar cab ride. A supermarket lay a ten-minute walk away.

Strategies for achieving these goals included the following:

Keeping our life as simple as possible through establishing and maintaining a routine suited to Pat's needs. Dementia sufferers don't like change.

Finding places and spaces, inside and outside the house, where I could attend to my needs.

As a morning person, I put a lot of attention on meeting

Pat's needs in the first part of the day.

Keeping Pat as healthy and well fed as possible, finding food she enjoyed and using my limited culinary skills to best advantage.

Ensuring I had all the necessary paperwork in place and keeping notes on Pat's condition to brief the medical people with whom we dealt. I had power of attorney over Pat's affairs and medical consent. Pat had made her will, but did not specify her last wishes. Based on my experience with Pat, I drew up my last wishes and lodged them with my will.

I remained sensitive to Pat's moods and tried to foresee them — without a great deal of success. I looked for patterns in her behaviour and strove to anticipate her needs. In 2011, I entered short accounts of Pat's condition in a day diary.

On June 3, I wrote, "Pat very good all day." On August 17, the diary entry read, "Confused, weeping in morning. But fine rest of day — quite delightful. Stroppy at bedtime. Delayed going to bed."

The notes I made on Pat's condition and the diary entries have proved invaluable in writing this book and have given me a sense of what life was like while I cared for Pat. Looking over them, I realized that I achieved the goal of keeping our life as normal as possible — most of the time. I carried in my head the positive and negative aspects of life with Pat. Almost up to our last day together, the former far outweighed the latter.

I did a SWOT (Strengths, Weaknesses, Opportunities, Threats) analysis to determine how best to implement the strategies. Strengths were pretty much the same as assets. I built on them as needed. The major weakness was my impatience, my desire to get things done as quickly as possible. Everything you do for and with a dementia sufferer takes twice as long as you expect. As I got Pat ready to go to a doctor or to have her hair done, I would joke, "The next job I'm applying for will be with NASA. Compared to getting you ready for an appointment, putting someone on Mars will be easy."

I kept an eye open for opportunities that would please Pat. She enjoyed yard-saleing. When the Unitarian Church down the street held its annual yard sale, I took Pat there and let her freely wander around the tables.

Threats included the ever-present one that Pat, in her weakened state, would fall and hurt herself. She did this several times, but I was nearby and helped her to her feet. I ensured that everything in our condo unit remained in the same place and that floors were clear of obstacles. Pat moved a box in one room and it was me who crashed to the floor. Fred, who lived downstairs, heard the noise and came upstairs to see if I was all right. We made only one modification to our home, installing a bar in the bathroom to make it easier for Pat to lift herself from the toilet. Pat being Pat, she seldom made use of it. The weather presented other threats, with dark, cold winters and dreary, wet summers often making it hard to leave the house. Pat was terrified of falling, even when I was holding her. Fortunately we had a couple of open winters, with little snow and milder than usual temperatures, while I was caring for Pat.

Keeping Pat Happy

I devised a wide range of tactics to ensure Pat's happiness. They included the following:

Meals and medications at the same time each day. I have an acute sense of time, something Pat always lacked and that did not improve during her dementia. Among the constant questions she asked me was "What's the time?" I see that now as a response to boredom.

Plenty of hugs!

A fixed bedtime.

The same plates and cutlery at meal times.

Always calling Pat "love" and "sweetheart" and "sweetie" as I had done in the past and always being polite with her — except when I blew my cool. I felt it better to have a number of small explosions rather than one really big one.

Telling Pat where I was going when I left the house — for groceries or to get money from the bank or a haircut. I hugged and kissed her before leaving and on my return. I checked with the home support workers about how Pat was during my absence. They almost inevitably reported, to Pat's last day, that she had been fine and no trouble.

Telling Pat how wonderful she looked. Pat said of a photo of a woman in a book, "She's beautiful." I said, "So are you. And you will always be beautiful to me."

Smiling and being cheerful at all times.

I would do and say silly things to keep Pat happy. She may not have understood my jokes, but the expression on my face and my body language obviously reached her and she laughed at them. At the supermarket, I would grab a shopping cart, turn to Pat and say, "Hop in and I'll drive you home."

One year we had mice and called in the pest management people. I explained to Pat how they operated: "When they hunt tigers in India, they tie up a goat and sit in a tree to wait for the animal to appear. Here they hunt mice by tying down a piece of cheese and sitting on top of a cupboard with their little mouse guns."

I put on one of Pat's hats and told her, "It looks better on you than on me." Pat laughed and said, "I don't know." Whether my clowning behaviour reached Pat, I never could tell. But it helped me to retain my sanity.

I talked to Pat about our travels together. As she took apart a map of Rome, I recalled our visits to the city and the time she gave the driver the finger. When I mentioned Carcassonne, her eyes lit up, and she enjoyed hearing about the night the rabbits danced near Croy. Again, how much she actually understood I never could tell. But these memories comforted her — and me.

When Pat went into care, I provided the institution with a list of her medications, her allergy (penicillin) and details of her condition. A military maxim claims, "No plan survives first contact with the enemy." And my plan for caring for Pat did not always survive changes in Pat's behaviour and moods. But it helped me to establish priorities, make decisions, identify the limits of what I could do for her, set boundaries and search for ideas and experiences that could make her life — and mine — as easy as possible.

I derived insights from quantum mechanics. Depending on how it is observed, an electron can behave like a wave or a particle. Thus, if you change the setting and the environment of a person with dementia and the way they are treated, their behaviour and condition will alter. I heard of a man with dementia receiving one-on-one care who shed ten years of his life. Placed in an institution, he went rapidly downhill. Pat always had one-on-one care, except for the time she spent in the Berkeley while I was in hospital and in the nursing home.

The Buddhist concept of the world being made up of the real and the unreal helped in caring for Pat. Sometimes she was with me, at others in a place I could not reach her. I tried to enter this world. If she said someone was stealing her things, I'd assure her that he or she would bring them back. If Pat said she wanted to go back to England, I did not dismiss the idea. I'd say, "Well, you'll have to get a passport" or "Where will we live?"

A woman with dementia demanded, again and again, to go home. The family filled a suitcase with her clothes, took her out the front door of the house and brought her in through the back door, telling her, "You're home now."

I was strongly influenced, and heartened, by Viktor Frankl's *Man's Search for Meaning*. He survived three years in Nazi concentration camps and prisons, developing the concept of logo therapy to explain his survival and that of others. It focuses on helping people to find meaning in life by creating a work or doing a deed, by experiencing something or encountering someone who inspires you to greater efforts and by learning how to deal with unavoidable suffering. You focus on what is worth doing rather than lamenting about your situation, reflect on what you have experienced and learned, find ideas, knowledge and wisdom wherever you can, share what you know and maintain a positive attitude to life. As Nietzche put it, "He who has a why to live can bear any how."

Pat was my why.

But I recognized that I had to have another why in my life, access to a world separate from caring for Pat, an arena where I could do my own thing.

Taking Care of Jim

While taking care of Pat, I continued to write books, completing four of them. *Canada's Forgotten Arctic Hero* told the story of George Rice. The Cape Bretoner served on the Greely expedition and died seeking food for his comrades on this ill-starred venture to Northern Ellesmere Island.

Disaster at Dieppe covered the futile attack on the French port on August 19, 1942, which cost the lives of almost a thousand Canadian soldiers and sent two thousand more into German captivity.

I spent the summer of 1963 in Dawson City in the Yukon as the last of the big gold mining companies was winding down its operations. *The Gold of the Yukon* tells what the community was like in the early sixties and of the old-timers in the Klondike, convinced that one day they would strike it rich.

The Moral Equivalent of War owes its title to an essay the American philosopher William James wrote in 1910. He asked how the comradeship, discipline, courage and self-sacrifice that emerge in wartime can be directed at fighting poverty, injustice and other ills of the world. My book looked at the various panaceas about community and human development that have emerged in the post-war years and described how James's concept was being implemented in Canada, Wales, England and Lesotho in Southern Africa.

Each weekday morning I arose at 5:30 a.m., washed, shaved and went to the Tower, the gym at Saint Mary's University, now the Homburg Centre for Health and Wellness. Here I exercised for forty minutes (weights and exercycle), showered and came home around seven, feeling refreshed. Pat usually slept while I was away; she had never been a morning person. In April 2010, I started doing vinyasa yoga with Stefanie

Winters, a gifted instructor. On December 21, 2011, I had a nirvana moment during yoga, a feeling of blissful nothingness. Exercise and yoga proved invaluable in maintaining my stamina and spirit while keeping me healthy.

Before I left for the gym, Pat would sometimes awaken and become fearful about my absence, asking again and again, "How long will you be away?" At other times, she would say, as once she did, "Have a good workout." I went to the gym on Sunday morning, devoting Saturdays to clearing up mail and paying bills.

On Wednesday and Saturday afternoons, beginning in November 2009, I took three-hour respites. I could have taken ten hours each week but preferred to be with Pat. She became somewhat disturbed when first I went on respite but soon adjusted to the routine. After making lunch, I left at one o'clock and headed for my bank on Spring Garden Road, Halifax's busiest street. Before doing my banking, I relaxed with a newspaper and a free cup of coffee; I figured I was paying the bank for it, somehow. Then I headed for Back Pages, a second-hand bookstore owned by Mike Norris, whom I had known since he started his business. A gifted artist and a thoughtful individual, he always had something of interest to discuss, as did Graham Lavers who looked after the shop while Mike was absent.

I struck up casual friendships like these at the gym. Dennis, Wendy, Greg, Lillian, David, Roy, Steven (a fellow writer), Doug and others offered a sympathetic ear as I talked about Pat and showed their concern for me.

Sometimes I would head for Barrington Street and lose myself in John Doull's disordered bookstore that contained many treasures — if you could find them! I spent a lot of time in the library. Here and in the bookstores I haunted,

I met old friends on the shelves and made new ones, helping to keep my mind alert while bringing back memories.
Books consoled me, opening up vistas on wider worlds than
the narrow one in which I lived while caring for Pat. I read
James Joyce's *Ulysses* twice, once to be able to say that I had
read it, the second time to enjoy this great, wordy, rambling
account of a day in the life of Leopold Bloom.

A Day in Our Life

I had the strong impression that Pat fought her dementia.
Her strong and resilient spirit that I loved and admired
sustained us both. She would try to write. I found a copy of
The Haligonians with the following notations opposite the
cover page, as if she was trying to make sense of the title: *H:
Hall: A: lanng on...*

In our last two years together, Pat seemed more relaxed,
less anxious and fearful, more content than she had been
during the early stages of her dementia when she had
spoken of jumping off a tall building or drowning herself.
This is a common feature of the late stages of dementia. We
had upsets and meltdowns but I know that Pat sensed the
presence of a loving and reliable person as her health deteriorated. She continued to care for me as I did for her; once,
in the kitchen, she made sure that I did not bang my head
on an open cabinet door.

Each day, when I returned from the gym, I would help Pat
out of bed and serve her breakfast before settling at my desk
for three or four hours, drafting outlines or typing manu-
scripts. Wanting to be near me, Pat would hover — another
feature of people with dementia — around my desk. I usually

ignored her, but sometimes she annoyed and distracted me from my writing. I would tell Pat, "I love you deeply and dearly but you are being a pain in the ass." Steering her into the living/dining room, I left her to "potter" — her word — until lunchtime. She seemed quite happy doing this.

After lunch I sat in the living room, reading a newspaper, magazine or book, keeping an eye and an ear on Pat. I have very poor eyesight, but very acute hearing and this helped me to keep track of Pat's movement.

Pat removed pieces of bread from the package and laid them out on the kitchen counter. This puzzled me. Telling her the bread would go stale, I put the slices back in the package and placed it on a high shelf where Pat could not reach it. I found her in the bedroom one day, dismantling the bedside lamp. I took it away from her. She did not resent this, nor my action with the slices of bread.

The mystery of Pat's interest in them emerged when I saw her, completely absorbed, placing pieces of toilet paper on the dining room table. I realized that she was recalling the time she made beautiful quilts with scraps of cloth. The memory of doing this persisted and gave Pat comfort.

Pat's other focus of attention was on newspapers, magazines and books, part of the world in which she once worked. The feel of them in her hands, the sight of words obviously comforted Pat. She would spend a whole afternoon "reading" a newspaper or absorbed in a book or a magazine or even a journal with empty pages; sometimes she read books upside down. She did not accept my offer to read to her but asked me for a pencil with which she marked up newspapers and magazines. I brought fashion magazines home from the gym. Pat delighted in some, ignored others.

Pat had a particular attachment to the illustrated edition

of Laurie Lee's *Cider with Rosie* and her books on cats. "I love that," she said of *Church Cats*. The Yellow Pages engaged her attention for hours. She pointed to an ad showing a man, telling me, "That's my father." She scanned the cover of Evelyn Waugh's *Vile Bodies* before throwing it across the room. John Grogan's *Marley and Me* suffered a similar fate. Pat liked the cute dog on the cover, but became angry on reading that it was "the world's worst dog." There had never been a bad dog or cat in Pat's life.

These actions showed that Pat's mind was still working, as did a charming incident when she picked up a paperweight from my desk. It had the face of a cat impressed upon it. Pat spoke to it and placed it on a windowsill so that it could see the garden.

Pat hung on to *La Femme Après 30 Ans*, a book that contained photos of sophisticated, soigné women. Joan Dawson, a friend, wrote of Pat, "Elegance — how impressive she was, with her distinctive style and poise, that could have passed in the most élite Parisian salons!" Did this book recall the days when she was well dressed and well groomed? By November 2010, Pat had lost all interest in her appearance. She wandered around our home in our daughter's high school cardigan, old, torn slacks and one of my jackets or in a dressing gown and underwear. We lived in a house filled with books and magazines, and Pat obviously found comfort in their presence on the shelves. Late in her dementia, she began to take books and magazines apart, tearing out pages. Much as I love books, I never tried to stop her doing this for it seemed to give her pleasure.

Until late 2010 we went for a walk every day. On Tuesdays and Fridays we did the groceries and on Saturdays we yard-saled. On Sundays, we walked to Point Pleasant Park, a favourite spot of Pat's, and visited the ducks in Quarry Pond, just inside its entrance. Pat greeted every dog she met and talked with the owners. In time, Pat could only manage a walk around the block. I had to coax her into doing this by telling her that we might meet Marcus, a big friendly Bernese that loved Pat.

Dementia sufferers need routine and links to the past.

The mother of a friend developed dementia. Living in the country, she hired local women to care for her. They had grown up with her and knew her ways. One made a special cake for her and asked her how she liked it. "I've seen better," came the reply. As my friend put it, "My mother would never have said that before her dementia." Caregivers secured large sheets of paper on which the woman wrote poems she remembered from childhood, illustrating them with drawings.

People with dementia never cease to amaze you!

The Globe and Mail of January 25, 2013, discovered the ability of people with dementia to recover elements of their former lives and put a name on it: "A new school of thought on dementia: Montessori principles aim to reduce anxiety and provide meaningful activity for adults with cognitive diseases." The piece dealt with a programme at L'Chaim Retirement Home in Toronto. A retired cardiologist sorted through cardiograms, a woman made cookies.

We always had our flu shots but kept medical procedures to minimum. In January 2011, I took Pat to the Maxillofacial and Oral Surgery Clinic. She became upset when the surgeon approached her with a needle to freeze her gums. I was called in and decided to cancel the surgery. The alternative to freezing Pat's gums was to sedate her and this might have had serious side effects. Everyone at the clinic was kind and helpful but even Pat's brief time there made her robotic. She stood in the hospital foyer, completely out of it, while I called a cab. She was fine when we reached home.

It is important for caregivers to stay in control of the medical procedures offered or given to those with dementia. This is the message of the PATH programme.

I decided it was better for Pat to live with non-threatening conditions than risk medical interventions that might have unfortunate outcomes.

The highlight of Pat's life, before and after she developed dementia, came from biweekly visits to her hairdresser, Ethel Sears. She had followed her around the city since arriving in Halifax in 1973. Ethel loved doing Pat's hair. Her care and attention to it, and to Pat, proved to be one of the best therapies for dementia.

Home care workers expressed amazement that Pat stayed on her feet for so long. "Must be all that walking," one said. Pat had problems with her feet stemming from a common problem of working-class people in Britain: poor quality or ill-fitting shoes. My father, an ex-soldier, insisted that my brother and I look after our feet and we always had good footwear.

I trimmed Pat's fingernails, but could not tackle her toenails or the calluses on her feet. A friend recommended Marcienne Mason, a registered nurse who ran Toe to Sole Foot Care. She did a splendid job caring for Pat's feet. She would work on them as Pat screamed bloody murder, even when Marcienne was not touching her feet. At the end of the session, Pat would thank her. I told Marcienne she should get danger pay. She laughed. "I have one patient who has to be held by two of her family while I do her feet." She'd tell Pat, "Thank goodness you have only ten toes."

Marie, Pat's sister, sent her a pair of moccasins. They proved ideal as Pat's ability to walk declined and she shuffled round the house.

During the summers and falls, Pat would sit on the steps in front of our unit, sometimes with the mouse from the computer she no longer knew how to operate. From time to time she would wander around the front garden and climb on a wall at the side of it. I kept an eye on her while she was outdoors and hastened to help her down. A Chinese woman helped me once. I explained, "My wife has dementia." Pat retorted, "I do not!"

I always cared for Pat with the belief that, whatever was happening in her mind, her emotions remained intact and she was capable of understanding something of the world around her. Dementia, however, messes up circadian rhythms. The routines I developed to care for Pat enabled us to get through the days, but other dementia sufferers wander around their homes at all hours of the day and night. Pat experienced "sundowners," a common phenomenon of those with dementia. As day wanes and light fades, they become agitated, confused, restless, abusive, out of control. These episodes may last for a short or a long time. Pat had a few of them but they passed very quickly.

After a simple supper, we settled down to watch TV. I looked for DVDs, videos and programmes that Pat would enjoy. This proved to be a hit-and-miss business. I thought she would like *The Music Man*, with its romantic plot and Robert Preston as the bold and brassy con man, but Pat showed no interest. She expressed delight when we found a DVD of *Charlotte's Web*, a book she loved, at a yard sale. The movie bored Pat. Peter Ustinov, as Poirot in *Dead Man's Folly*, kept Pat's attention, as did episodes of *Monarch of the Glen*, which may have stirred memories of our time in Scotland. *Avenue Montaigne* tells of a naive young woman who comes to Paris, finds a job in a bar and meets three interesting neighbours. Pat sat through it, perhaps because it was in French, a language in which she was fluent. Or she may have empathized with the shy young woman adapting to a new setting. Pat laughed at slapstick and spoofs and argued with Rameses II when his face appeared during a programme on the pharaohs. Pat talked to the TV: "You should have known that! That's disgusting!" During *Hotel Babylon*, a British series, a character ran a bath. Pat followed suit, but did not get into it.

My experiences with watching Pat watch TV made me realize that she really enjoyed some programmes, even in her time of severe dementia. Iris Murdoch loved watching *Teletubbies* on TV, a somewhat bizarre children's programme on the BBC featuring strange small characters who squeaked and did odd things. Did TV programmes remind Pat of pleasant times in the past, like those she had had in France and Scotland?

We always went to bed at or before ten o'clock.

I was blessed in that Pat usually slept well. Caregivers need their sleep, and I was able to rely on several hours each night of undisturbed repose. Pat seldom left our bed. When she did, I had no trouble coaxing her back to it. In 2011, Pat did not go to bed in the evening, preferring to sleep on the couch or in her chair. Sometimes I would, with great difficulty, lift her up as we both laughed and got her to bed. At other times I left her where she was. When I arose for my early-morning pee, I would try to get her to bed and usually succeeded.

Once or twice Pat fell out of bed. She would laugh as I helped her back into it, assuring her that she had not damaged the floor. As in the past, we spent some of our best times in bed, contented and relaxed, holding hands. I stroked Pat's cheeks as we enjoyed the simple pleasure of just being together and at peace.

I do not seek to minimize or downplay the difficulties of caring for Pat, this woman I had been so lucky to marry and to love for so many years. We had good days and dreadful ones, weeks that proved surprisingly normal and others when I felt that I was going crazy, shouting and swearing at Pat. I longed to walk out of the house, grab a plane, go somewhere, anywhere, to be away from the person I loved more than anyone else in the world. Even my devoted care and our deep and enduring love for each other could not defeat the disease eroding Pat's mind as her health declined.

I managed to keep Pat at home, in Thorndean, the old house she loved so much, until her very last day, as the last act of my beloved wife's life unfolded.

Music

Music can comfort dementia sufferers and is also being used in cancer treatment, pain management and end-of-life care. When the husband of a friend, an avid baseball fan, developed dementia, she hired a music therapist who played "Take Me Out to the Ball Game" on her guitar. His face lit up with delight.

Music stimulates the ventral tegmental area (VTA) in the brain. This pleasure centre, linked to motivation and reward, can also be stimulated by chocolate, cocaine and love.

Pat and I loved classical music, especially opera, which we saw in New York, London and Rome. While at Manchester

University, I appeared with Covent Garden Opera as a super. In *Turandot* — "Awful old bitch," the director explained — I played the role of the executioner. As a soldier in *La Bohème*, marching across the stage without my glasses, I almost fell into the orchestra pit.

When DesGrieux, the hero of Puccini's *Manon Lescaut*, first sees the heroine, he sings, "*Donna non vidi mai.*" I would tell Pat that it reminded me of the first time I saw her, translating it as "I ain't never seen a better looking broad than you."

Pat introduced me to the bel canto operas of Bellini and Donizetti and to chamber music, which became my lifelong passion. I shared with Pat my large repertoire of rude and bawdy songs. If she sighed "Oh, dear," I'd sing,

> *Oh, dear, what can the matter be?*
> *Two old ladies locked in a lavatory*
> *The first maid's name was Elizabeth Humphrey.*
> *She went there to make herself comfy.*
> *They've painted the seat*
> *And she can't get her bum free.*

When the stress of caregiving threatened to overwhelm me, I'd retire to the kitchen, dance around it with an imaginary partner, talk gibberish and sing, "Life presents a dismal picture,/Sad and empty as the tomb." After a few minutes, as Pat looked on completely bewildered, I'd say, "No point in having two crazy people in the house," and return to my normal behaviour.

Around the time Pat developed dementia, CBC FM (now Radio 2), changed its programming to cater to a younger demographic. Instead of wall-to-wall classical music, the station featured caterwauling, vocally challenged singers and the monotonous riffs of jangling guitars. I searched for CDs to please Pat. She appeared to be consoled by what I found, listening for ninety minutes to Verdi's *Requiem*, telling me that she remembered Elgar's *Chanson du Matin* from her childhood, humming along with *Greensleeves*, *Jealousy* and the music of Bach. Before Pat developed dementia, we watched an enjoyable production of Mozart's *The Magic Flute* on TV. When the Queen of the Night aria came on the radio one evening, Pat danced her fingers on the table to it. In early 2011, she shushed me when I tried to talk to her. Completely entranced, she was listening to Marietta's lovely aria from Korngold's *Die tote Stadt*.

Oscar Wilde claimed that "music is the art which is most nigh to tears and memory." Pat could recall the hymns of her youth and liked one of my songs, to the tune of "The Church's One Foundation:"

> *We are the Royal Air Force, a jolly lot are we,*
> *We cannot fight, we cannot shoot, we cannot do PT.*
> *We go to church on Sunday and sing with all our might:*
> *'Per Ardua ad Astra,' bleep you, Jack, I'm all right.*

She enjoyed the songs of Ivor Novello, especially "Rose of England," sung by a beery baritone, and the deep voice of the Australian bass-baritone Peter Dawson; she sang "Waltzing Matilda" with him. She remembered the rude words put to the Dvorak's "Humoresque:" "Please refrain from urination while the train is in the station./Or you will be peeing on the line." And the British kid's version of "The Toreador Song" from *Carmen*: "Toreador, don't spit upon the floor,/Use the cuspidor. That's what it's for."

Music helped to keep up my spirits, confirming the observation of Cervantes: "He who sings scares away his woes." Returning from the gym in the morning, I would sing to myself, *sotto voce*, "The Road to the Isles" and long to take it again.

Back at home, I would look at Pat and other songs would course through my mind: "So in Love," from *Kiss Me Kate*, which we saw in London, and "If Ever I Should Leave You" from *Camelot*." It ends, "No, never would I leave you at all." And, always, in Pat's last years, the voice of Walter Huston singing "September Song:" "And these few precious days I'll share with you, These golden days I'll share with you."

Meals

Pat and I spent our adolescence in wartime Britain when food was rationed; we never saw a banana or other exotic items. Our attitude to food reflected the north/south divide in that country. Northern diets such as scouse, the dish that gave residents of Liverpool their name, feature lots of carbo-hydrates and meat. Geared to heavy industrial work, the food gave northerners strength and stamina. We ate to keep up our strength, dismissing lettuce as "rabbit food." Salads and such-like fancy foods would weaken you, as they did effete southerners. And pasta? That Eyetalian stuff? Never!

Before I married, I had the typical careless bachelor attitude towards food: You eat to live, not live to eat. In the Arctic you need about five thousand calories a day to sustain yourself and lots of fat to ward off the cold. On Arctic expeditions I acquired this nutrition in a rough and ready fashion. On the ice shelf in 1959, my diet relied on large quantities of C and K rations left over from the Second World War. On Operation Hazen, Geoff Hattersley-Smith, the leader, put a lot of thought into the food. Breakfast consisted of porridge with lots of butter, supper of a stew into which was pitched anything we had at hand. Brian, my tent mate, added cheese to the mix one evening. The result tasted awful, but we ate it. In between these meals, and on the trail, we relied on soup, shortbread bars, chocolate and other delicacies. Despite the squalor in which we lived, with caribou hairs from the skins under our sleeping bags finding their way into the food, no one got sick.

Pat loved her grub and had much more refined tastes than I did. She claimed she had not cooked before we married, that her mother was a religious cook: everything she served was either a sacrifice or a burnt offering. Pat introduced me to the delights of Caesar salad, spaghetti carbanaro, lasagna and other dishes. I was always amazed at how she managed to get all the ingredients of a meal on a plate and on the table at the same time, something I had difficulty doing when I took over the cooking. Pat kept her family well fed while working full time. As food editor of *Atlantic Insight* she prepared special dishes or assigned articles on them; you cannot run a recipe in a magazine or book unless someone has made it.

Quite suddenly, despite her love of cooking, Pat stopped making our main meal in 2006. Jane Buss, former executive director of the Writers' Federation of Nova Scotia, delivered excellent meals over one winter. Recognizing my complete incompetence as a cook, we relied on Meals on Wheels and frozen specialties from the Victorian Order of

Nurses for our one main meal of the day. At first Pat seemed to enjoy the deliveries. Then, quite suddenly, she began to leave large parts of the food uneaten. With my dislike of waste and desire to please Pat, I looked around for packaged food she would enjoy and we established a routine. I became a reasonable cook if the instructions on the packages were clear. I prepared fish, potato patties and peas for one meal and served up pasta, soup and salad. Breakfast always consisted of fruit and yogurt, plus toast and marmalade. Sometimes Pat responded to the first offering with "Yum," at other times with "Yuck" and often by asking me, "What is this?" In evenings we had rolls with ham, beans on toast or scrambled eggs on toast, the last item the only one in my original culinary repertoire. Pat greatly enjoyed it. I later broadened my scope of cooking by making poached eggs on toast. I always had oatmeal cookies on hand, but had to ration them after Pat consumed almost a whole package one morning.

I tried to liven up the meals by joking with Pat. She enjoyed a cup of coffee a day and once asked me for half a cup. "Top half or bottom half?" I asked. Pat laughed and said, "Whatever is best." I would apologize if I gave her the wrong spoon for her ice cream: "Hope you don't mind." And we laughed. Pat greatly enjoyed ice cream. Once, when I offered her it, she said, "I have no money." These words recalled Pat's early days in a family short of money.

I learned to give Pat one item of food at a time. Otherwise she came up with bizarre combinations. The salad would end up in the soup, the ice cream on the pizza. I found a photograph stuck between two pieces of bread.

As Pat's dementia worsened, so did her eating habits, and meals became very messy. Sometimes she would eat her meals quite calmly, sometimes with her fingers, at others she pushed away the plate. This upset me because I was concerned about ensuring that she was well fed. Pat usually ate what I offered her after a delay of a few minutes.

One of the saddest things as a caregiver was seeing Pat, who had made such wonderful meals for her family, and with whom I shared so many during our travels (including the cassoulet we failed to finish in Carcassonne), slowly losing interest in what she once so much enjoyed — even ice cream.

This, alas, is one of the common features of severe Alzheimer's.

Continence/Incontinence

These two words loom large in the lives of caregivers with the ever-present possibility that one will turn into the other. When that happens, you reach a breaking point and realize that the care of the loved one is beyond you, more than you can handle. It's a terrible but inevitable time, when a person with dementia loses control of bowel and bladder. Incontinence is one of the signals that indicate that he or she must go into care. Either that or you must prepare yourself for a very messy life.

I was very fortunate that Pat remained largely continent during the time of her dementia, although there were occasional lapses with which I managed to deal. Through the clairvoyance of love, I became attuned to Pat's need to go to the bathroom. Elderly gentlemen like me have to relieve themselves during the night. I turned this nuisance into an opportunity. Waking at two or three in the morning, bent on going to the john, I would find Pat alert and restless.

Reading the signs, I helped her out of bed and half-carried, half-walked her to the bathroom. I knew she needed her own time there. A stock of humour books kept up my spirits while I waited.

They included ones by the Two Ronnies, Ronnie Corbett and Ronnie Barker, whose absurdist dialogues suited my mood:

> *The Noise Abatement Society and the Kennel Club have joined forces to produce Hush Puppies.*

> *The longest ever swearing-in ended…this afternoon after 6½ days when the witness, Bert Ormsby, instead of holding the Bible and reading the card, held the card and read out the Bible.*

Schoolboy howlers recalled British traditions of political incorrectness:

> *Q. What are rabies and what would you do for them?*

> *A. Rabies are Jewish priests and I would do nothing for them.*

And a book of anecdotes about Sir Thomas Beecham, who stated,

> *There are two golden rules for an orchestra: start together and finish together. The public doesn't give a damn what goes on in between.*

When I heard the toilet flush, I'd go into the bathroom to ensure that Pat washed her hands, joking, "We don't want the Black Death starting here." Sometimes I had to be forceful about this ritual. At other times, Pat's face would light up and she would tell me how nice it felt to have her hands in warm water.

Pat usually went to the bathroom on her own during the day, almost to the end of her life. She needed my help at times, saying afterwards, "You are a splendid person" or "It's nice to have you with me" or thanking me.

I mistimed Pat's needs once. Waking up in the early morning, I found her lying with arms and legs in the air, like an upturned turtle. The sheet was wet, but a large plastic bag I had placed under it had kept the mattress dry. I hurried Pat to the toilet and quickly changed the sheet.

Pat's incontinence proved to be episodic.

She peed herself in August 2010 and a few days later, saying, "I smell." And sat on a chair in the dining room and had a crap. I cleaned up and sprayed perfume over the site. I didn't like the scent, but it was better than the other smell.

But Pat's bathroom habits followed the usual pattern and I had no more problems with them until December 2011. One day I could not find her. I located her just inside the front door, gazing contentedly into the street, crapping into a wicker basket. I roared with laughter and took her to the bathroom. If I saw Pat heading for the front door with a certain expression on her face, I'd intercept her and take her to the toilet.

A cab driver told me about his mother who had Alzheimer's. She died at ninety, after fourteen years with the disease, her last four years spent immobile in bed, unable to speak and incontinent. I realized how lucky I was with Pat. Only at the very last did she become incontinent and have to suffer the indignity of wearing diapers.

Caregiving

Most caregivers are members of the immediate family of the sufferers and keep them in their own homes as long as possible. In Nova Scotia, this costs the government $33 a day, compared to $300 a day in long-term care outside the home and around $1,000 in hospital. It's easy to see why governments are promoting home care even as families struggle with the demands made upon them.

I had no idea how to proceed when I became Pat's main caregiver. I saw looking after her as a duty, a way of honouring our marriage vows, an expression of my passionate love for her. I fumbled badly in my efforts to make life as comfortable as possible for Pat. There are plenty of guidebooks on caregiving for people with dementia, but a lot depends on the kind of life you had before it struck. I brought to my new role all I was capable of, physically, mentally, emotionally, financially, yet too often found that this was not enough to keep Pat happy. And I realized my total dedication put my own physical and mental health at risk.

In times, I felt trapped, while at the same time reluctant to hand over care for Pat to strangers. A woman looking after her husband with cancer and Alzheimer's finally agreed to have a home care nurse visit him: "You have to let them in, because you're going to explode." Of the free time the nurse's visit gave her, she said, "It's a double-edged sword. All the time you're thinking, 'I hope everything is all right.'" I never worried about Pat when I went on respite. I assumed that home support workers would have no problems with her and inevitably they reported that she had been fine. We hired these workers after Pat was diagnosed with end-stage Alzheimer's in October 2009. Before that, I was Pat's sole caregiver, learning as I went along, adapting as best I could to her moods and behaviours. I discovered that when nothing was happening when I was not with Pat, something was happening. Several times she turned on the taps in the bathroom sink and almost flooded the place. One day, she put a book in the oven. Peter, our grandson, came for lunch and switched it on without looking. The result was a new version of the cliché about cooking the books. I realized that some of the bizarre behaviour that Pat demonstrated, moving around, hiding and rearranging things, represented an effort by her to have some control over her confused world. Actions that appeared illogical to me, putting Parmesan cheese into a coffee cup, may have been a memory of what Pat had once done when she cooked.

From November 2009 to early 2012, we hired home support workers from the Canadian Red Cross Home Partner Service at just over $10 an hour for six hours a week. That was as long as I wanted to be away from Pat. In all we had twenty-four workers. They ranged from one who came into the living room, flopped into a chair and reached for the newspaper to a control freak. She kept an eagle eye on everything Pat did. When I arrived home, Pat was trying to escape from the house. This individual gave me a valuable piece of information: "Alzheimer's patients don't like water." This was certainly the case with Pat who gave up having her daily bath during the severe stage of her Alzheimer's. The worker did manage to wash Pat and to change her clothes. But I phoned the Canadian Red Cross and told them, while this lady might be just the right person for some clients, she was not a good fit with Pat.

One of the most difficult aspects of caregiving by non-family members is finding individuals who connect with sufferers. Empathy, compassion, understanding and a gift for caring are more important in this respect than formal courses. The curious and complex chemistry of human relationships can aid or inhibit caregiving. I heard of a woman with dementia placed in a room in a nursing home with another sufferer. Neither knew the other, but the new arrival decided the other woman was her sister. She accepted the role and they did everything together. The buddy system has great potential in caregiving.

I have almost no memory of the majority of the home care workers who looked after Pat while I was on respite. Most just sat or watched TV with her. At first, Pat looked distressed when I left the house. As she became accustomed to the routine and knew I would return, she adapted to my absences.

We were blessed with three workers to whom caring was a calling not a job. Angela, the first to arrive, brought treats for Pat. After her first visit, she wrote, "Nice lady. Very polite husband. Patricia slept entire time. Got up once to go to the bathroom. Good shift." in the client log (November 28, 2009)

Before leaving the house, I told Pat that the visitors had come to keep her company, not to look after her. It was important to respect Pat's need for independence.

Paul, a young man with innate gentleness, had lived in the Yukon and Central America. When I returned from respite, we chatted about the north. He told me of Pat's engaging curiosity about what was happening in the street and the books she perused. He quickly gained Pat's affection and she reciprocated it. Paul wrote in the client log, "Pat was excellent today; happier and interested." (January 9, 2010) and "Excellent visit; had a stroll in the garden and picked flowers." (May 29, 2010).

Tracy, an energetic young woman, wanted to do more for Pat and me when she came. Several times she cleaned the bathroom and kitchen floors, although I never asked the workers to do household chores. Tracy developed a wonderful rapport with Pat, who always looked good and relaxed when I came home from respite. Sometimes they would stand on the front porch to greet me on my return. As Pat's feeding habits deteriorated, her clothing became incredibly messy. Tracy was the only worker who could persuade Pat to change them. She gave her a sponge bath writing in the client log, "She really doesn't like being undressed but having her things prepared ahead speeds up the process and lessens the frustration. Pat seemed in better spirits afterwards." (January 25, 2012).

When I worried about Pat peeing the bed and soaking the mattress, Tracy suggested putting a large plastic bag on top of it. This worked well when the inevitable happened.

The care given by Angela, Paul and Tracy were balm to my troubled soul as I continued to do my best for Pat and to look after her as well as they had.

Chapter Eight
The Last Act; Losing Pat

The last act is tragic, however happy the rest of the play is.

Blaise Pascal

I watched, helplessly, as Pat's life ebbed away through 2011. As she slept, her breath came heavy and forced, and I wondered if she would awake or just slip away from me one night. I felt I had only skin and bones in my arms when I hugged Pat, her face wrinkled, skin shrivelled, the flesh on her arms as loose as a garment sleeve, hands skeletal.

Do we know when death is near, when our end is imminent? Pat told me of "The Battle of Otterbourne," in which a Scottish warrior, about to go into battle, foresees his death:

But I hae dreamed a dreary dream,
Beyond the Isle of Skye:
I saw a dead man win a fight,
And I think that man was I.

During the First and Second World Wars soldiers going into battle told their mates that they did not expect to survive, that their number had come up. Almost inevitably they were proved right.

A story from what is now Iraq tells of a servant who goes to the market in Baghdad. He returns, terrified, and begs his master for his fastest horse. "Why do you need it?" the master asks. "I met Death in the marketplace. I must flee to Samarra tonight," the man replies. The master gives the servant his swiftest horse and the man speeds to Samarra. The master then goes to the market where he meets Death. He has no fear of him because he knows his time has not come. The master upbraids Death for scaring his servant. "I'm sorry," says Death. "I did not intend to do that. I was just surprised to see him in Baghdad. I have an appointment with him in Samarra tonight."

Did Pat know how little time we had together? On August 20, 2010, she said, "I believe I am dying." In October of that year, Pat told me, "You can live without me." During 2011, she moved, slowly, relentlessly, towards her appointment in Samarra. In March, at the Dalhousie Dental Clinic, she said something about being "at the end of my life." Around this time I had a dream. Pat and I are in an elevator. It ascends, stops and Pat gets out. I stay on it. It descends to ground level and I set out in search of Pat. I cannot find her, staggering along a muddy, potholed road, helping a small boy (myself when young?) over gaps in it. Did my dream foretell

Pat's ascent to heaven and the rough time I would have after her death?

The Barrier

Caregivers, sooner or later, break and hit the Barrier, the point where, physically and emotionally exhausted, they can't go on. The Barrier resembles the Wall that runners hit when they reach the limits of endurance and can go no faster. Sometimes you feel you are on a slippery slope, about to fall into an abyss. To avoid hitting the Barrier or ending up in the abyss, you grab on to anything that gives you a grip on reality. The process is spiral, not linear. You sense yourself losing your grip on your sanity and whirling downwards. Suddenly, something happens and you are moving upwards again, feeling reassured and a little light headed over some small, trivial incident.

Our last year together, 2011, proved to be the best and the worst of times since Pat developed dementia. I had become fatalistic, believing what would be, would be, and that I could not stop Pat's progress into deeper and deeper dementia. Over the winter of 2010–2011, I suffered from cabin fever, even as Pat proved easier to care for as she became more relaxed and content, a feature of the late stage of dementia. We had upsets from time to time, especially when Pat refused to take her medication. I stopped giving her Alendronate for her osteoporosis. When I put drops in her eyes, she said, "You are the best."

Time and again, I slid down the slippery slope or saw the Barrier coming near, felt I could no longer care for Pat. Then she would make some small gesture, tell me she loved me, smile, call me sweetheart. My spirit soared and I would renew my determination to do all I could for Pat's happiness and comfort.

When Paul, exceptionally good with Pat, left one day, he held out his hand. Pat took it, leaned forward and kissed this gentle young man on the cheek. One day Tracy arrived, upset and weepy after being hassled by her agency. Pat went to her, put her arms around her and consoled her. As Tracy put it, "She's still a person. A lovable person."

One day in May 2011, she said to me, "I'm happy with you."

A few weeks later, while I was checking a reference, Pat messed around with parts of a manuscript I was working on. I became angry. Pat threw papers at me. In a maniacal mood, I grabbed her, cuffed her gently around the ears and pushed her out of my study. Looking up from my desk a few minutes later, I saw Pat peering from the door opposite with a wonderful kind and loving look. I rushed over to her and we embraced and kissed with a passion I had not known for many months. Pat said, "You're the only person in this place…" She left the sentence unfinished, but I knew exactly what she meant. Pat pottered around the place, quite happily, for the rest of the morning.

She still wanted to go back to Britain to see her parents. And her sense of humour still remained. Pat laughed when I told her, after she knocked over a glass of water on the dining room table, that she was "very economical. You made a small amount of water go a long way." I spied an ant in the kitchen and told Pat, "That's an ant. If it's a female and has relatives, it could also be an aunt." She laughed.

On June 17, as I was leaving for the gym, Pat, lying in bed, held her hand out to me. I took it and we kissed.

Twice Pat said, "I love you." I wrote in my diary, "There is something remaining of the relationship we once had. Some small, flickering flame. But how do I keep it alight?"

I took Pat to a nearby drugstore for blood work, the first time she had been outdoors for months. She managed the walk there and back without difficulty.

Pat became increasingly sensitive to my moods. Once, when she became upset, she assured me, "It has nothing to do with you."

In June, for the first time, Pat expressed no delight when I told her that she was going to have her hair done. The process of shutting down had begun.

Shutting Down

I had managed to avoid hitting the Barrier or sliding into the abyss, even as I wrote, in early May, "caring for Pat becomes an impossible burden at times and she becomes the butt of my frustration." Pat's eating habits became erratic and I had to cut up her food for her. She awoke early one morning, sat on the edge of the bed, then stood by the radiator in my study. I asked her, "Is there anything you need?" She replied, "Practically everything." From time to time, she knew she was Pat Lotz, but Thorndean was not her home.

When Anne West and Sally came by in July, Pat ignored them, going into the bathroom and the kitchen. Anne commented on how frail she looked. Pat crept around our home without slacks or panties, sat with her head in her hands and smelled awful. On July 11, she asked me, "Who are you?" I decided I needed a few weeks away from her: "One of the hardest things is that, no matter how much you love someone, no matter how powerful that love, there is very little you can do to help that person as they sink deeper and deeper into dementia. The further and further into dementia Pat goes, the more I feel I love her and want to take care of her."

Pat talked a lot to herself and muttered words I could not understand. In late July, I arranged for Pat to go into a nursing home for seven days, the only length of time available. I laughed when I received the entry forms from the home. They wanted Pat to bring seven pairs of pyjamas with her. Pat had not worn these or changed her clothing for months. I cancelled the booking, believing that looking after Pat for seven days would be less trouble than dealing with the bureaucracy at the nursing home. I wrote, "Pat is not hard to manage, except when she goes to the john at night." I put flowers from the garden in a vase and Pat thanked me for them. She continued to "read" and take apart books, magazines and newspapers. On July 26, I wrote, "I know I can do little for Pat, but she is in familiar, safe surroundings, pottering away during the day and seemingly content while crying from time to time — less so in recent weeks. The positives of being with Pat far exceed the negatives."

In August, we hit another snag after I noticed that Pat's right eye had filled with blood. I still remember the panic on the face of the ophthalmologist when he examined the eye. He told me that Pat had a large ulcer, caused by a virus, in it. He could not operate on it because Pat was taking Warfarin, a blood thinner. She could go blind in the eye, which is what happened because she resisted the eye drops I tried to administer. Curiously, this loss of vision did not seem to bother Pat as she knew her way around our home.

In the same month as her eye appointment, home support workers gave Pat a bath and changed her clothes so she looked and smelled a whole lot better.

In September, I had a dream in which Pat came to me, bright, eager and beautiful as once she had been. In another dream I pushed her to the ground.

Eating became messy, with food ending up in Pat's clothes, on the floor and in the bed when I fed her there. She expressed appreciation when I took her to the toilet one night, then asked me, "Do you know where my husband is?"

On one frustrating evening, I hustled her out of the bedroom then invited her back and we hugged and were close again. I kept asking myself as the Barrier and the abyss loomed nearer: How much longer can I cope with Pat's behaviour? How can I create spaces and places for myself? What's the best thing to do for Pat, for me?

In October, Pat had no interest in going to Ethel's to have her hair done, but I managed to persuade her to make the trip. One morning in that month, as we lay in bed, holding hands, I felt our love to be as strong as ever. A day or so later, returning from the gym, I gave Pat her usual hug. She called me to her and gave me a hug of her own volition. I noted, "Almost like old times." These wonderful, lucid, loving moments kept me going.

In the following month, I developed a twitch in my right cheek and nearly hit the Barrier. Pat became restless in bed at night, talking without making any sense. Somehow, despite this, we managed to communicate for I knew Pat so well and did not need words. She thanked me for feeding her and giving her medications and said she was sorry if she upset me.

In December, when Anne West and Sally visited, Pat sat on the couch, head bowed, a copy of C. S. Lewis's *Miracles* in her lap. She ignored Anne but obviously enjoyed the attention Sally paid to her. Roma Arsenault also visited us, commenting on how small Pat had become. Pat paid no attention to Roma while she was with us. When she left, Pat very graciously thanked her for coming and said she hoped to see Roma again.

By now, Pat ate all her meals with her fingers and created a unique dish, bacon ice cream, when she put one in the other. She made patterns with her spoon on placemats, perhaps a memory of making quilts by cutting up cloth. As Pat could no longer make the trip to her hairdressers by taxi, Ethel came to our home with a device to clean her hair. When she explained how it worked, Pat said, "That will be wonderful."

As we entered the new year, I became edgy, awaiting the results of a colonoscopy, which showed nothing amiss. I said, "Oh, dear" over and over as Pat once had until she told me to stop.

Pat's sense of humour remained intact. After giving her breakfast in bed, I brushed crumbs off her T-shirt, saying, "Don't want you looking crumby." She laughed.

Tracy, a home support worker, helped Pat to change her clothes, something I could never do. She was surprised that Pat was still on her feet and going to the toilet on her own at this stage of her dementia. She now spent every night on the couch or in her chair, with no strength to lift herself up and out of them. I did not force her into bed. Checking on her one morning at two thirty, I discovered she had taken off her slacks and that her legs were ice cold. I put her slacks back on, a pillow under her head and blankets over her. In the evenings she no longer watched TV with me but sat at the table or on a chair.

She was eating very little and sleeping a lot, sure signs that her life was ending. I refused to recognize this. Life with Pat was increasingly difficult, but I still preferred to be with her than with anyone else in the world. Paradoxically, as Pat drifted further and further away from me she also seemed to come closer. On February 4, 2012, Pat told me how grateful she was for what I was doing for her. I noted in my diary, "Excellent day! Almost like normal."

Pat's death lay only nine days away.

The End of Pat's Pilgrimage

I believed, wrongly, that Pat's indomitable spirit and my love would give us a few more years together. Her death came with dramatic suddenness.

I had extended my respite on Saturdays to four hours to have a meal out after I had given Pat her lunch. On Saturday, February 11, I came home to find Pat sitting on the floor of our bedroom, a blank expression on her face. Sharon, the home support worker, told me that she had fallen and paramedics were on the way. They arrived, checked Pat's vital signs, asked Sharon and I questions, strapped Pat to a stretcher and took her to the Halifax Infirmary Emergency Department. I went with them. We waited in a corridor until a room became available. Pat looked and sounded fine, chatting away without making any sense. I stayed with her while she was settled in bed and went home. The hospital phoned me at 7:40 p.m. Pat was resisting being examined. Could I come in and be with her for a while? I returned to the hospital, held Pat's hand, calming her down. An X-ray showed nothing broken, but it was decided that she should spend the night in Emergency. Leaving Pat sleeping peacefully, I left the hospital just after eleven in the evening on a dismal, rainy night that matched my mood.

Awakening the following morning, feeling desolate without Pat beside me in bed, I headed for the hospital to retrieve her. With the considerable help of Lisa, the discharge nurse, I dressed Pat and called a cab.

Farce mingled with tragedy on our journey home.

The cab driver, a large man who overflowed the front seat, told me, "I don't walk." Without help there was no getting Pat into the house. At Thorndean, I dashed out of the cab to open the door, only to find the lock frozen. As was the back door lock. Fortunately, Bonnie and David, our upstairs neighbours, were at home. I pushed frantically on their bell and they came down to help me. David unfroze the front door lock then helped me to carry Pat into our home. We had a tug-of-war with her at the cab. David thought I was trying to put her into it. Pat shouted and screamed as we carried her into the house but settled down once she was in bed and slept for the rest of the day.

The hospital had put diapers on Pat, the first time she had worn them, and given me a bag of them for future use. I thought I could continue to care for Pat if I could change her diapers.

But I finally hit the Barrier.

Pat fought me as I changed her diaper. Anger welled up in me as I realized how incompetent I was in doing this simple task. I knew she would have to go into care. I swore at Pat, abused her verbally and physically in my berserk mood. When I left for the gym on the morning of February 13, Pat was asleep. On my return I changed her diaper, again cursing my incompetence. Pat bore my reproaches stoically. She now seemed to be out of it in a way that had never happened before. It was obvious that she had pain in her legs. I called Dr. Swinemar, who suggested I take Pat to Emergency.

Again the paramedics came and I drove with them to the Halifax Infirmary. We waited in a corridor for a room to be available. I held Pat's hand and kissed her. She gave me one last, beautiful smile before being wheeled into Room 15. I went to the Continuing Care Department to fill in the forms for Pat to be admitted to a nursing home. Someone made vague mention of a person from Internal Medicine coming to see me about "admission." Presumably this meant placing Pat in a long-term care bed.

Back home, I mooned around the house until seven thirty in the evening when Dr. Weltus, the Emergency Department physician, called me. Could I come to the hospital? Tired, not having eaten all day, I told him I'd come in tomorrow. Then came the chilling response: "There may not be a tomorrow." Waiting for a cab in the cold, made even colder by my grief, one thought pulsed through my mind: "Pat, my beloved wife, is dying."

At Emergency, Dr. Weltus told me that Pat had suffered two seizures and that another X-ray had shown multiple fractures of her pelvis. They had been missed on the previous scan because of the difficulty of placing Pat, who struggled strongly, on the machine. She also had a bladder infection.

Dr. Weltus sat on one side of Pat's bed with me on the other.

"Are you saying Pat is dying?" I asked him.

"I don't have a crystal ball, but…"

Struggling to breathe through an oxygen mask, her body heaving, Pat obviously had little time to live. She had been catheterized, was receiving antibiotics to deal with the bladder infection and narcotics for the pain from her fractured pelvis. A monitor registered respiration and heartbeat, which was surprisingly strong. "It's because of the pain," Dr. Weltus explained, adding that they were doing all they could to keep Pat comfortable and to ease her pain.

She was not going gentle into that good night.

Dr. Weltus said she could be gone in five minutes or two days.

He asked me if I had eaten and suggested I go to Tim Horton's for a snack and a coffee.

Hearing is the last sense to go before death. Before I left Room 15, I whispered into Pat's ear, "I loved you from the moment I saw you and I love you still." Around eleven, I headed for Tim Horton's, numbed with grief, had a dutchie and an orange juice and went back to Emergency. A frantic man rushed towards me, calling my name. I knew what had happened.

Pat's pilgrimage through life had ended and she was finally at peace, no more doubting, no more questioning, no more uncertainties. My beloved wife had gone out in characteristic style. "She fought to the end," Dr. Weltus told me.

The monitor was disconnected, the tubes removed and I was left alone with Pat. We had been married for fifty-two years, two months and a day. My beautiful, bright, shining wife had left me. In her place lay a shrivelled husk, hair tangled, skin sallow, eyes closed, mouth open in the rictus of death. I kissed them, hugged the lifeless body. With an empty heart I walked through the empty midnight streets to an empty home.

I received two accounts of Pat's death. The Medical Examiner Certificate gave the cause as "Complications of Pelvic Fractures due to fall." Other significant causes were dementia and hypertension. The manner of death was reported as "Accident." A report from the Halifax Infirmary to Dr. Swinemar identified Pat's presenting complaint as general weakness, the diagnosis as urosepsis and the departure destination as morgue.

On the afternoon of February 16, I went on my last date with Pat. I put on a clean shirt, new slacks, my best jacket and my Canadian Executive Services Organization tie, in memory of the book that Pat and I had written together. Pat lay in an open casket, serene and beautiful, hair neatly done; I quite expected her to open her eyes, look at me and say, "Hi, sweetie! Let's go home." I kissed her cold lips three times then walked into a world and a life without Pat. Had she survived the fall, the infection and her other ills, Pat would have spent what was left of her life in a long-term hospital bed, comatose, in pain, catheterized, alone.

Anne West described Pat's swift passing as "God's grace." And no one deserved that more than my beloved wife, that enchanting, spirited person who so enriched my life and those of so many others.

On September 8, a group of Pat's women friends gathered to pay a tribute to her, an Old Broads' Brunch. They produced a bookmark for the occasion with two photos and a summary of Pat's qualities on it: "Life Long Learner; Courage and Grace; Sense of Humour; Kind to every Living Thing; Rich in Spirituality and the founder of the Old Broads' Brunch."

Below Pat's photos were the words "Fondly remembering a gracious hostess, a wonderful friend, and a beautiful woman."

To this I could have added, "And a wife with whom I had a lifelong love affair that transcended dementia."

And so the journey of Pat's pilgrim soul ended. But not quite…

Envoi

Though lovers be lost love shall not; And death shall have no dominion.

Dylan Thomas, *"Death shall have no dominion"*

Death does not end a loving relationship.

Pat left me with the legacy of her love for me and a wealth of memories of the magical moments we shared.

We are atop a high hill on Mull, entranced by the stark beauty of the rugged land around us.

We are wandering the silent streets of Rome in the freshness of early morning after throwing our coins into the Trevi fountain.

We are on the West Bay Walkway in Victoria, reveling in the sunlit day, watching the birds and the planes taking off from the dappled waters of the inner harbour.

A clerk in a bookstore told me after Pat died that she had

often seen us out walking: "Your love for each other just shone from you." At the end of our life together love was all we had — and all we needed for a happy life in those last years.

Pat is not dead while her story comforts and consoles others, telling them how to deal with dementia with courage and grace, as she did.

> *Nor shall Death brag thou wander'st in his shade*
> *When in eternal lines to time thou grow'st:*
> *So long as men can breathe, or eyes can see,*
> *So long lives this, and this gives life to thee.*

Bibliography

There is an enormous amount of literature on dementia and it grows apace every year. Most of the material falls into two categories: prescriptive accounts, which tell readers what to do while caring for those with dementia and personal ones, tales of caregiving. In *Pilgrim Souls* I have attempted to blend the two.

The provincial branches of the Alzheimer Society have material (brochures, books, videos) on the disease and other forms of dementia. And there are doubtless many websites that I did not consult. As a caregiver, you can get too much information and lose your common sense.

I found the following helpful in understanding dementia and caring for Pat:

Bayley, John, *Iris: A Memoir of Iris Murdoch*, London, Abacus, 1999.

Geist, Mary Ellen, *Measure of the Heart: Caring for a Parent with Alzheimer's*, New York, Springboard Press, 2008.

Genova, Lisa, *Still Alice*, New York, Gallery Books, 2009.

Goffman, Erving, *Stigma: Notes on the Management of Spoiled Identity*, New York, Simon and Schuster, 1963.

Gray-Davidson, Frena, *The Alzheimer's Sourcebook for Caregivers* (3rd. ed.), Los Angeles, Lowell House, 1999.

Gregory, Richard L. (Ed.), *The Oxford Companion to the Mind*, Oxford, Oxford University Press, 1987.

James, Oliver, *Contented Dementia*, London, Vermilion, 2008. (The SPECAL website is www.specal.co.uk)

Joordens, Steve, *Memory and the Human Lifespan: Course Guidebook*, Chantilly, Virginia, The Great Courses, 2011.

Lindner, Robert, *The Fifty-Minute Hour*, New York, Bantam, 1954. (This book has been reprinted several times, once in 1999.)

Mace, Nancy L. and Peter V. Rabins, *The 36-Hour Day* (5th ed.), Baltimore, The Johns Hopkins University Press, 2011.

Menzies, Heather, *Enter Mourning: A Memoir of Death, Dementia and Coming Home*, Toronto, Key Porter, 2009.

Munro, Alice, *Away from Her*, Toronto, Penguin, 2007. (The title story was originally called "The Bear Came Over the Mountain.")

Rockwood, Kenneth and Chris MacKnight, *Understanding Dementia: A Primer on Diagnosis and Management*, East Lawrencetown, Pottersfield Press, 2001.

Sacks, Oliver, *The Man Who Mistook His Wife for a Hat*, New York, Summit Books, c. 1985.

Sacks, Oliver, *Musicophilia; Tales of Music and the Brain*, Toronto, Vintage Canada, 2008.

Other Sources

Through the courtesy of Dr. Laurie Mallery, I secured a copy of *PATH Clinic: Palliative and Therapeutic Harmonization*, subtitled "Team-based Assessment and Care Planning." This very valuable guide to dementia and caregiving should be more widely known. Dr. Mallery also embodied the principles of caring into her amusing book *The Salami Salesman and His Daughter Falafel* (Bloomington, Author House, 2011), which tells how she, her sister and her mother cared for her frail and dying father.

The Alzheimer's Project is documented in three DVDs and a book. Sponsored by HBO, this material presents stories of people with dementia and their caregivers and an overview of the research being done on dementia. The book, published by Public Affairs, New York, in 2009, subtitled "Momentum in Science," deals only with the research. Chapters focus on scientists studying personality traits that may play a role in preserving brain function, the story of the Sisters of the Blessed Virgin Mary in Dubuque, Iowa, and how their lifestyle appears to inhibit the development of Alzheimer's, the role diet and exercise plays in lessening the chances of developing dementia, the immune system, the impact of hereditary (a study of seven siblings, only one of whom is not developing dementia), drug developments and more.

The book offers a useful clarification on dementia: "People often use 'dementia' and 'Alzheimer's disease' interchangeably, but the two words do not mean the same thing. Dementia describes a cluster of symptoms from a loss of cognitive skills — thinking, remembering, and reasoning — that is so severe the person has trouble carrying out daily activities. Dementia is usually caused by a disease or a condition…"

Alzheimer's, now known as AD, is a disease that inevitably causes progressive dementia.

Marcia R. Seitz-Ehler, public affairs specialist at the U.S. Consulate General in Halifax, very kindly sent me a copy of the National Alzheimer's Project Act, which became law on January 4, 2011. It states that the term *Alzheimer's* means "Alzheimer's disease and related dementias." Among other things, the act focuses on early diagnosis of AD and the coordination of care and treatment of citizens with Alzheimer's and calls for the establishment of an advisory council on Alzheimer's research, care and services. Heavy emphasis is placed on reporting and the evaluation of federally funded programmes. The project contains a sunset clause. The hope is that by December 31, 2025, AD and other dementias will be curable.

Ms. Seitz-Ehler also sent me a copy of the *National Plan to Address Alzheimer's Disease*, issued by the U.S. Department of Health and Human Services. It deals with preventing and treating AD by 2025, enhancing care quality and efficiency, expanding support for people with AD and their families, enhancing public awareness and engagement and improving data to track progress. It notes that receiving twenty-four-hour care in a nursing home in the U.S. is estimated to cost $78,000 a year. Nearly half (48 per cent) of nursing home residents have AD. The early onset of AD can now be detected through imaging and biomarkers in brain, blood and spinal fluids, which makes early diagnosis much easier. Special attention is paid to building a workforce with the skills to provide high-quality care, and mention is made of the need to encourage providers to pursue careers in geriatric specialties. The U.S. already has a geriatric academic career awards program.

Nineteen states and a handful of local entities have published plans to address AD. Clinical trials are taking place for drugs that might cure or alleviate AD and studies are being done on behavioural interventions such as exercise. In the year 2010, 1,393 projects were being undertaken on AD and related dementias.

At the time of this writing (March 2013), no cure has been found for Alzheimer's and other dementias, so there will be continuing emphasis on developing ways of caring for those suffering from them.

Acknowledgements

I am most grateful to Heli Anderson for her comments on the draft of the manuscript and to Pat Langmaid, Jill Robinson, Betty Moore and Dr. Ross Ainslie for sharing their stories of dementia with me.

Our daughter Fiona and our grandson Peter, computer whizzes, gave me valuable support in finding the information I needed when I needed it.

The more you write, the more you need skilled editors. I would like to thank Melissa Churchill and Chelsey Millen for making the book more readable, and all those at Formac Publishing involved in the production of *Pilgrim Souls*.

Jim Lotz
July 11, 2013